GW00372967

ARTHRITIS & RHEUMATISM

by John Cosh MD FRCP

To my wife, Kit in appreciation of
her loving support over so many years.

Published by
Amberwood Publishing Ltd
Park Corner, Park Horsley, East Horsley, Surrey KT24 5RZ
Tel: 01483 570821

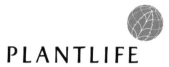

PLANTLIFE

The Natural History Museum, Cromwell Road, London SW7 5BD

Registered Charity No. 328576

Amberwood Publishing supports the Plantlife Charity,
Britain's only charity exclusively dedicated to saving wild plants.

ISBN 1-899308-17-2

Typeset and designed by
Word Perfect, Christchurch, Dorset.

Cover design by Howland Northover

Printed in Great Britain

CONTENTS

About the Author

For over twenty years the author was a consultant physician and rheumatologist in Bath, on the staff of the Royal National Hospital for Rheumatic Diseases and the Royal United Hospital. He had also previously trained as a cardiologist while a University Lecturer in medicine at Bristol Royal Infirmary. His special interests in Bath included a study of the course of rheumatoid arthritis as observed and treated from its beginning, studies of the involvement of the heart in the rheumatic diseases, and the development of thermography in the measurement of inflammation and its response to treatment. He published many papers on these subjects and was later the author, with Dr J R Lever, of a book on "The Heart in Rheumatic Diseases".

After his retirement in 1979 he was associated for ten years with the work of the Bristol Cancer Help Centre, developing an interest in complementary therapies with particular relevance to cancer.

Acknowledgements

The illustrations in this work are reproduced with the kind permission of the Arthritis and Rheumatism Council for Research, Registered Charity No 207711. The Publishers also wish to thank Mr G. James, Medical Artist at the Bristol Royal Infirmary, and Professor M.I.V. Jayson of the Rheumatic Diseases Centre, University of Manchester.

Note to Reader

Whilst the author has made every effort to ensure that the contents of this book are accurate in every particular, it is not intended to be regarded as a substitute for professional medical advice under treatment. The reader is urged to give careful consideration to any difficulties which he or she is experiencing with their own health and to consult their General Practitioner if uncertain as to its cause or nature. Neither the author nor the publisher can accept any legal responsibility for any health problem which results from use of the self-help methods described.

Introduction

All of us at some time suffer from bodily aches and pains or stiffness, and if these complaints are at all persistent we may well refer to them as our "rheumatism". Fortunately most such symptoms settle down with a little care and simple treatment. But persistent pain and swelling in one or more joints – arthritis – is a more serious matter and may in the course of time become disabling. Rheumatism and arthritis are common problems worldwide, irrespective of climate and temperature.

In Britain rheumatic complaints are the commonest cause of visits to the doctor, responsible for one fifth or more of attendances. In addition, we deal with many such complaints ourselves without troubling the doctor, treating them with remedies from the pharmacist or the health food shop. And increasingly today people are turning to the therapies of complementary medicine.

Age is an important factor. Rheumatic complaints, particularly osteo-arthritis, increase with age, so that the growing proportion of older people in our population means that the nationwide burden of rheumatic complaints is growing.

As a major cause of absence from work, rheumatism and arthritis are a heavy cost to the community in terms of loss of earning and productivity and in the cost of medical care. The leading example is back pain. In the year 1991-2 it was responsible for the loss of 80 million days of work with a total expense to the community estimated at £6 billion. As for the frequency of osteoarthritis, it has been found that 60% of people over 65 years of age have moderate or severe osteoarthritis in one or more joints.

The word "rheumatism" doesn't have any exact medical meaning: it is an inclusive term, generally meaning any kind of musculo-skeletal complaint. This could involve muscles, tendons and their sheaths, ligaments and connective tissue (non-articular rheumatism) or pain and inflammation in joints themselves (arthritis) of which there are a number of forms and causes. The total number of different rheumatic disorders that have been medically identified is about 200.

Without going into too much detail we can set out the most important forms of rheumatic disorders as in Table 1, which follows the order in which they will be described in this book.

Group	Condition
Non-articular rheumatism	Soft tissue rheumatism
	Back pain and disc lesions
	Special problems in shoulder, hand and foot
Degenerative	Osteoarthritis
Inflammatory	Rheumatoid arthritis
	Similar forms of polyarthritis
	Childhood forms of polyarthritis
	Ankylosing spondylitis
Connective tissue disease	Polymyalgia rheumatica
	Systemic lupus
	Scleroderma (systemic sclerosis)
Crystal arthritis	Gout and pseudogout
Bone disorders	Osteoporosis
	Rickets and osteomalacia
	Paget's disease

Table 1: Classification of rheumatic complaints

The relative frequency with which different rheumatic complaints occur in Britain can be judged by the result of a review made by the Royal College of General Practitioners. They asked GP's to note the frequency with which their patients presented with rheumatic problems. Their findings are shown graphically in Table 2. We see that back pain is by far the commonest complaint (45%), followed by osteoarthritis (21%) and non-articular rheumatism (15%).

Back pain	45%
Osteoarthritis	21
Non-articular rheumatism	15
Rheumatoid arthritis	4
Shoulder problems	4
Knee problems	2
Gout	2
Others	7
	100%

Table 2: Frequency of rheumatic disorders seen by GP

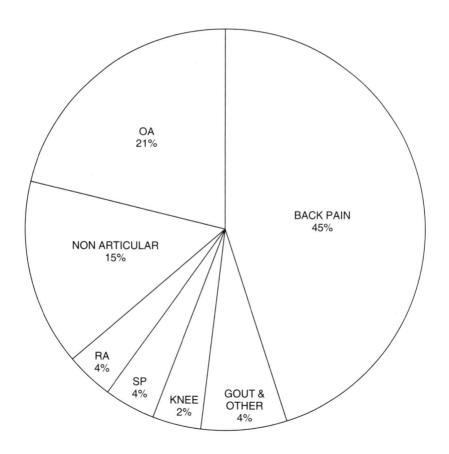

1 | Soft tissue rheumatism

Soft tissue rheumatism is the name given to a variety of complaints affecting tissues other than joints. This means muscles, tendons and tendon sheaths, ligaments, bursae, and the fibrous connective tissue which separates all of these structures.

The cause of these troubles is usually some form of injury, stress or misuse, perhaps by accident or perhaps by thoughtless action on our own part. We may be at fault in our posture or in the way in which we make everyday movements or actions. In some forms of soft tissue rheumatism there may be complications due to pressure on or injury to a nerve. This can cause additional symptoms such as numbness or tingling in the area served by that nerve, or weakness in the muscles that it controls.

The result is usually pain, stiffness and difficulty in movement and sometimes swelling. Unpleasant though these symptoms may be they do not undermine our general health, as some kinds of rheumatism may do. Even so, persistent discomfort and difficulty in movement can have a distressing effect on our well-being through interfering with our daily activities.

Fibrositis

Fibrositis is the name rather loosely used to mean pain, tenderness and stiffness in the fibrous connective tissue beneath the skin and between muscle layers, and possibly in the muscles themselves. It most often affects the side of the neck or the region of the shoulder girdle where there are powerful muscles supporting the shoulder blade and arm. Or it can affect the side of the trunk or the back. The name suggests that there is inflammation ("-itis") of fibrous tissue, but there is little proof of this. It probably arises from unusual or repeated muscular stresses such as carrying heavy loads when our muscle aren't really equal to the task. Or perhaps we have fallen asleep with our neck or arm in an uncomfortable position keeping the muscles and tissues stretched. Exposure to cold or a draught makes things worse. Being immobile for a long period, say, when sleeping heavily always leaves us a little stiff, particularly if we are getting on in years; a few minutes stretching, moving and massage will soon put this right. But the trouble is more serious if there has been additional stress on muscles and exposure to cold, such as may happen if we fall asleep with the neck inadequately supported when travelling by car, coach or plane with a jet of air directed at us.

The treatment for fibrositis is with local warmth and firm massage. For prevention we must avoid excessive muscular stresses, protect our muscles from cold and see that our head and neck are properly supported when resting or sleeping.

Fibromyalgia

This is a condition in which there are many very tender areas and pressure points, usually over muscle masses, and tending to affect the two sides of the body symmetrically. Common tender points are over the neck muscle at the base of the skull, over the big trapezius muscle at the side of the neck, around the margins of the shoulder blade, and there are many others (see Figure 1.1). Firm pressure at these points makes the sufferer wince or cry out with pain. Yet there has not necessarily been any particular muscle stress or exposure to cold. Unlike the briefer discomfort of fibrositis, fibromyalgia pain and tenderness are persistent and are often associated with anxiety and depression. It is commoner in women than in men and may form an important part of the complex disorder known as *myalgic encephalomyelitis* (ME) or *chronic fatigue syndrome*. Although it may follow a viral infection such as glandular fever, this is not necessarily so. Fibromyalgia disturbs the normal pattern of restful sleep. Insufficient night-time rest leads to daytime fatigue, anxiety and tension, thereby setting up a vicious cycle.

The treatment of fibromyalgia is difficult. Vigorous forms of exercise and massage tend to make things worse. The psychological aspect calls for sympathetic support and counselling; some patients are sufficiently depressed to justify prescription of an antidepressant drug, although this can only be part of the treatment. Attention must be paid to daily

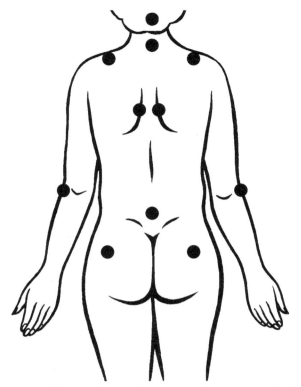

Figure 1.1: Fibromyalgia – Common tender points on the back

activities and life style, advising avoidance of tiring and stressful tasks, but encouraging activity which is within the patient's powers. Gentle physical treatment helps: this may include hydrotherapy and shiatsu, and correction of postural faults with the Alexander method.

Injuries

Serious injuries like fractures can have far reaching and long lasting effects on the body and may set the scene for the development of osteoarthritis in later years. Here we shall consider the less serious results of injury that can be called soft tissue rheumatism.

A heavy fall, whether or not we break a bone can cause extensive bruising due to the blow itself or to tearing of muscles in the limbs or trunk. Blood shed in this way in the tissues may track along between muscle layers or beneath the skin. It not only looks alarming but will also hamper movements, requiring a long period of patient treatment as the body's repair cells get to work to absorb and disperse the bruise. Too long a period of immobilisation for an injured limb, or indeed any part of the body, can lead to weakness and wasting of unused muscles which can take weeks or months to overcome. Co-operation with the physiotherapist will be needed in a programme of graded exercises helped by local heat, massage and possibly diathermy.

Sports injuries are a common cause of painful disability. Whatever the sport, it is important that we prepare for it with training and a warm-up period and look after our general physical fitness. The *skier* is at risk particularly from ankle injury and from falls. The *footballer* can easily damage a knee cartilage from a twisting injury or pull a hamstring muscle. The *cricketer* too can pull a hamstring muscle, or wrench a shoulder in bowling. In any sport *chest wall* injuries can result from a direct blow or from a violent twisting movement: these may result in a torn intercostal muscle which can be quite as painful as an actual fracture in a rib, seriously limiting deep breathing and body movements. The immediate treatment for a torn or bruised muscle is with direct pressure to limit further bleeding in the tissues, and with a cold compress. Ice packs are often used (including the convenient bag of frozen peas) but very cold packs should not be kept in place for more than a few minutes. In some cases an injection of long lasting local anaesthetic is needed. For chest wall injuries strapping is no longer used as it was found liable to cause congestion in the underlying lung.

The homoeopathic remedy arnica is widely used after bruising injuries. Either a small quantity of the tincture is added to the water of the cold compress, or the homoeopathic tablet is taken e.g. as a number of doses of the 6th potency at half hourly intervals.

Tendon injury

A torn or ruptured tendon is usually the result of a sudden violent pulling force, but a tendon may rupture easily if weakened by disease. The most striking example of rupture due to force is that of the Achilles tendon which transmits the power of the calf muscles to the heel bone in an action such as standing on tiptoe. It causes a sudden agonising pain and the actual "snap" will be felt and perhaps heard. A very similar injury in the lower calf can be due to the rupture of the less important Plantaris tendon which has a function similar to that of the Achilles tendon. Surgical repair is needed for an Achilles rupture, followed by a period of immobilisation in plaster and then rehabilitation.

Another common example is rupture of the tendon of the long head of the biceps muscle in the upper arm. This tendon runs up in front of and over the head of the humerus, and is attached to the scapula above the shallow socket in which the head of the humerus is held. This rupture usually happens in an elderly person due to friction weakening the tendon where it lies against the head of the humerus. The patient may feel the "snap", which can accompany quite a gentle shoulder or arm movement: some bruising later appears beneath the skin and characteristically there is a change in the shape of the biceps muscle when the arm is bent. As the muscle still has another head, attached to the coracoid process of the scapula, near the socket of the shoulder joint, it still functions though with less power, and no repair is needed.

Rheumatoid arthritis can weaken a finger tendon so that it gives way during normal use of the hand. The extensor tendon of the middle or ring finger may break, so that the finger cannot then be straightened (Figure 1.2). As the break is situated on the back of the hand, it is not

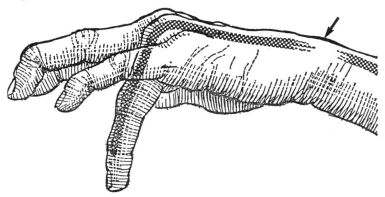

Figure 1.2: Ruptured tendon – The extensor tendon of the ring finger has broken at the point indicated. The finger cannot now be straightened.

difficult for the surgeon to repair it and restore normal movement. Less often a flexor tendon gives way, deep within the palm, usually affecting the middle or ring finger, which cannot then be flexed. Surgical repair is necessary, but it is technically more difficult than for the extensor tendon, and the result may not be so good.

Tendon sheaths

A number of tendons around the wrist and ankle are enclosed in a sheath right up to the point of attachment to a bone. The sheath's purpose is to allow free and frictionless movement of the tendon. Irritation and inflammation of the sheath (tenosynovitis) can be caused by unusual stress and overuse of the muscle in some repetitive action, which then becomes painful. A tendon sheath that is commonly affected is the one which extends (i.e. straightens) the thumb, on the back of the wrist (de Quervain's tenosynovitis). Treatment is by immobilisation with a light weight splint, and a cold compress in the acute stage, resting the arm in a sling. An accurately placed injection of a small dose of cortisone into the tendon sheath brings prompt relief.

Trigger finger

Repeated pressure on the centre of the palm, as may happen with the frequent use of a tool such as a screwdriver, may damage the flexor tendon of the middle or ring finger. The sheath becomes thickened and narrowed at the point of pressure and the tendon too is thickened, forming a nodular swelling. When the finger is flexed, the tendon nodule is pulled up, towards the wrist, through the narrowed place in the sheath. But when the finger is to be straightened again, the nodule cannot slip easily down again, and the finger remains flexed. It has to be pulled straight by the other hand. The small "snap" felt by the patient gives it the name "trigger finger".

Although annoying in its interference with finger movements, trigger finger is not painful. It can usually be cured by a well placed injection of cortisone into the sheath under a local anaesthetic. Surgery is rarely needed.

Bursitis

A bursa is a small sac containing a trace of fluid which acts as a protective cushion between moving parts of the body near joints or at pressure points. We have many of them, mostly only a centimetre or two in diameter, and we are unaware of them unless they give trouble through inflammation or injury. "Housemaid's knee" is the best example; the bursa here lies in front of the lower part of the knee cap and is subjected to pressure when we kneel on a hard surface (Figure 1.3). Another is near the point of the elbow, pressed upon when we lean on our elbows on a desk or table, and is often swollen in a person with rheumatoid arthritis. Another important bursa is near the shoulder joint, between the head of the humerus and the underside of the outer end of the collar bone. Others are found near the heel. Inflammation of any bursa is usually the result of chafing or undue pressure, especially with rheumatoid arthritis; it usually settles down in time with simple rest and protection, but recovery is quicker with a local injection of a small dose of cortisone. However, should the inflammation be due to bacterial infection antibiotic treatment would be necessary and cortisone would be harmful.

Tennis elbow

This gets its name because it can be caused by the repeated vigorous tug of the forearm extensor muscles in making a backhand stroke at tennis;

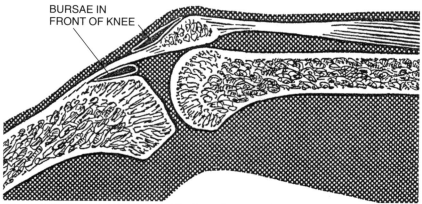

BURSAE IN
FRONT OF KNEE

Figure 1.3: Housemaid's knee – The bursa between the patella and the skin becomes inflamed and tender. A second bursa, behind the tendon, may also be affected.

any similar action can have the same effect. The forearm extensors, which straighten the fingers and wrist have a common attachment to the outer bony point of the elbow – the external epicondyle of the humerus. A sudden forceful pull can tear muscle fibres near the point of attachment. Repeated tears will prevent healing, resulting in a tender area of inflammation two or three centimetres from the epicondyle. Complete immobilisation would allow healing in time, but as this is usually impractical, an injection of local anaesthetic and cortisone is the usual treatment bringing relief within a day or two.

Carpal tunnel syndrome

A strong broad ligament runs across the flexor side of the wrist, lying deeply beneath the skin creases on that side of the wrist. It is attached to the forearm bones and its purpose is to hold in place the strong tendons which flex the fingers and wrist. The space in which they lie is the "carpal tunnel", and there is another important occupant in the tunnel, the median nerve. This nerve controls all the small muscles of the hand and also carries sensation from most of the palm and fingers, excepting the little finger and the neighbouring half of the ring finger (Figure 1.4).

There is no spare room in the carpal tunnel so that if anything causes swelling in the area, there is damaging pressure on the median nerve. The result is tingling and numbness in that part of the hand which the nerve supplies; in severe cases this is very unpleasant, with a burning character, disturbing sleep, sometimes spreading up the forearm. A sufferer may try and get relief by hanging the arm out of the bed at night. Causes of the swelling and pressure within the carpal tunnel include swelling of the wrist joints, due to arthritis, tenosynovitis, fluid retention e.g. at the time of the menopause, or with thyroid deficiency. If pressure on the nerve persists, the small muscles of the hand weaken and waste, which may become obvious in the muscles of the ball of the thumb.

In a mild case it may be sufficient to apply a light weight wrist splint and rest the forearm and hand, as much as possible in an elevated position. Usually the best treatment is a well placed injection of local anaesthetic and cortisone into the carpal tunnel. Should this fail, the surgical release of the constricting fibres of the ligament will relieve the pressure on the

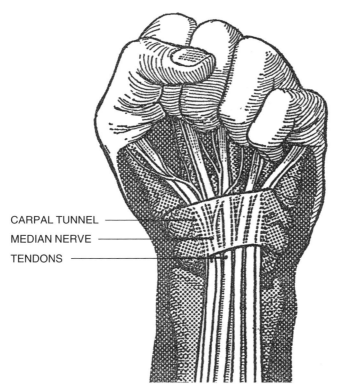

Figure 1.4: Carpal tunnel – The flexor tendons and the median nerve lie together beneath a broad ligament on the inner side of the wrist.

CARPAL TUNNEL
MEDIAN NERVE
TENDONS

nerve. The ligament heals afterwards, but in a more relaxed position so that the tendons are kept in place, and pressure on the nerve does not recur.

Repetitive strain injury

Under this heading are the many possible tissue injuries caused by overuse of a limb or hand in a frequently repeated action. Very often the subject maintains an awkward posture and lacks proper support for the limb – something which, with adequate forethought might be avoided. It is common in women operatives in assembling equipment on a production line working against the clock. In musicians trouble can arise from awkward positions e.g. of the left hand and wrist in a violinist, or in the thumb and fingers of a woodwind player. Overuse of individual muscles, uncomfortable postures and hunched shoulders give rise to muscle tension and fatigue, ligamentous strain and tenosynovitis. The situation may become emotionally charged if the worker is under pressure, making rest breaks difficult. Some cases give rise to litigation. Treatment usually means a break from work and appropriate physiotherapy. Prevention is most important, involving proper awareness of posture and ergonomic design of seating, bench, video screen etc.

2 | Soft tissue rheumatism (continued)

Low back pain

Posture. We are all familiar with aching and stiffness in the lower back brought on by a period of stooping over a heavy task. Relief comes from straightening up, resting the strained muscles in the lumbar region and some firm massage. To prevent this we must see that the work bench (or kitchen table, or ironing board) is at the right height for us, minimising the strain of work.

The key to the prevention of most lower back troubles is in our posture, whatever we are doing – sitting, standing or walking. The natural shape of our lumbar spine is slightly hollowed, and our diagram (Figure 2.1) shows the natural lumbar curve, or lordosis. If we can learn to be subconsciously aware of this we shall avoid much back discomfort. The same applies to the upper back and shoulder girdle and neck where we should learn to avoid an unnecessary stoop and hunched up shoulders. Correction can be taught by postural exercises, whether performed on our own or in a group. Here the Alexander method can be of great value.

Ligamentous strain is a more serious cause of low back pain. Heavy lifting work, especially if it involves a sudden strain may tear one of the many ligaments which bind together the vertebrae, either between their bodies or their bony projections (spinous and transverse processes) or around the facetal joints (Figure 2.2). The pain can be sudden and acute. It forces us to rest, if necessary by lying on a firm bed with local heat, massage and a pain killer. Sometimes the help of a physiotherapist is needed, with deep heat given by diathermy, and supervised graded exercises as we recover.

Disc lesions are the main cause of persistent low back pain. The intervertebral discs are firm fibroelastic pads lying between neighbouring pairs of vertebral bodies, having the important task of cushioning the

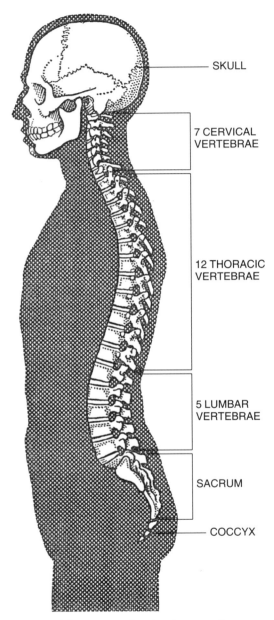

SKULL

7 CERVICAL
VERTEBRAE

12 THORACIC
VERTEBRAE

5 LUMBAR
VERTEBRAE

SACRUM

COCCYX

Figure 2.1: The spine – showing its natural curves

vertebrae against the vertical forces of weight bearing and the jolting they can receive when we walk or run.

Each disc has a relatively soft centre, the nucleus pulposus, ringed around by the harder annulus fibrosus; this is bound to the vertebrae above and below by the surrounding annular ligament (Figure 2.2). The discs bearing the greatest pressure are those in the lumbar region,

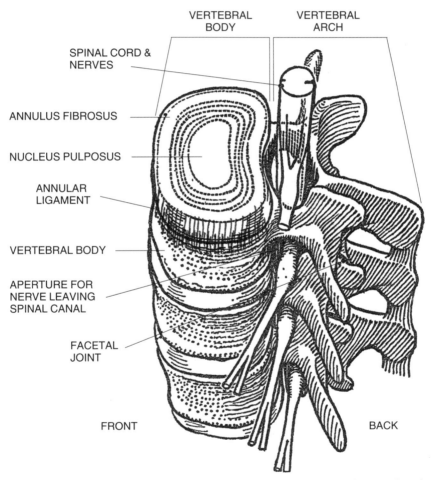

Figure 2.2: Lumbar vertebrae – showing the intervertebral discs, the spinal cord and the spinal nerves

particularly the lowest of all, between the fifth lumbar vertebra and the sacrum (lumbosacral). This is the disc most prone to damage.

An *acute disc lesion* begins with a tear in the annular ligament, usually caused by a sudden lifting strain made while bending forward. When we make such an effort with conscious preparation we tense the powerful lumbar muscles which support the spine. But in an unguarded moment we may not activate these protective muscles, and great strain is then placed on the annular ligament especially at the back, where it may tear. Not only is this extremely painful, but the combination of increased pressure on the disc may force disc material backwards through the torn ligament – a "prolapsed disc". The actual volume of disc material displaced can be quite small – little more than pea sized, but in the confined space of the spinal canal this is serious.

The spinal cord and the nerve roots springing from it lie within their protective membranes in the spinal canal. The spinal cord itself ends opposite the first lumbar vertebra. Below this the spinal nerve roots continue downwards emerging on each side between the vertebrae, forming the nerves which supply the lower limbs. Figure 2.3 shows what may happen if the disc prolapse presses on a nerve root near its point of exit between two vertebrae. This commonly happens at the level of the lowest (lumbosacral) disc, and the nerve root which suffers is the first sacral nerve, which is an important component of the sciatic nerve. This means that the sudden low back pain will be accompanied by pain transmitted by the compressed nerve root, perceived as pain coming from the back of the thigh and leg – sciatica. Less often the prolapsed disc is at one or two levels higher, in which case the pain in the affected nerve area will be in the thigh.

Treatment. The severe pain of an acute disc lesion demands immediate rest. This means lying flat on a firm mattress, either with a board beneath it or on the floor. Local heat and a strong analgesic are needed and will have to be repeated until the painful muscle spasm in the lower back has been relieved. Getting up for toilet and other purposes is a problem, best solved by the sufferer rolling on to his side and thence on to the floor, then carefully standing upright. Rest in this fashion may be needed for some days, but there are dangers in too long a period of immobilisation.

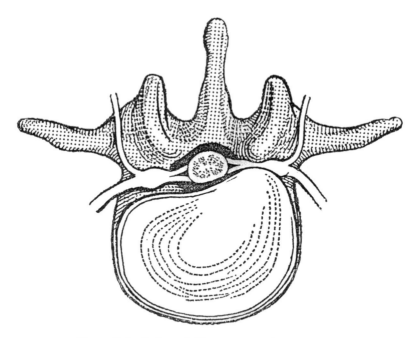

Figure 2.3: Prolapsed disc – compressing a nerve root

Under the supervision of the doctor or physiotherapist a programme of graduated movement and exercise is started; sometimes traction is helpful, either for brief periods or continuously over some days. Hydrotherapy can be valuable at this stage.

Most disc lesions heal naturally without the need for surgery. Care must be taken to avoid a recurrence. This means paying attention to posture when standing or sitting. The best seat is a firm one, giving support to the small of the back, with hips and knees at right angles, and arms to the chair to give assistance in standing up. The design of the car seat is important: most modern ones incorporate firm lumbar support. Great care is needed in picking up heavy objects. The patient must be taught the safe way of lifting i.e. bending at the knee, keeping the back straight, using the leg and thigh muscles to do the lifting (Figure 2.4). Walking is usually the safest exercise, always remembering to maintain a good posture.

Manipulation is not usually necessary, but if required should only be done by an expert, well after the acute pain has settled. Where needed it can help restore spinal mobility.

Surgery may be needed if simple methods fail and the pain and signs of nerve root pressure continue. The surgeon will need precise information on the site and size of the prolapse before operating. This can best be done with an MRI scan which obviates the previous method of X-raying after injecting radio-opaque material into the spinal canal (myelogram).

Osteoarthritis of lumbar spine (lumbar spondylosis) is a common cause of chronic low back pain and osteoarthritis is discussed in detail in the next chapter. It mainly affects older people and is usually the end result of long years of heavy physical work, possibly with disc lesions too - either past

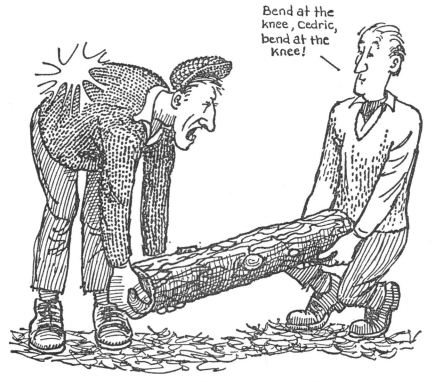

Figure 2.4: Heavy lifting – How not to do it!

acute lesions or more gradual degeneration of the discs. The cartilage in the facetal joints becomes worn and bony outgrowths develop in the line of the ligaments between the vertebrae. The result is much reduced mobility and pain and stiffness on movement. During a painful episode local heat, massage and physio or hydrotherapy will help and for a time a light weight supporting brace or corset may be justified. However, as far as possible, the accent should be on maintaining mobility and a good posture. Again, the Alexander method is of value.

Other causes of low back pain

Ankylosing spondylitis begins by causing pain and stiffness in the sacroiliac joints, characteristically in young men, though women too can be affected (see Chapter 6) It tends to be an indefinite ache, radiating down the back of the thighs, and as there is usually "nothing to show" it may be months before the diagnosis is recognised. Over the course of years this low grade inflammatory process may spread upwards throughout the spine which can become rigid. The emphasis of treatment is on maintaining mobility and preventing a forward stoop while anti-inflammatory drugs are given for the relief of symptoms.

Osteoporosis (see Chapter 9) begins painlessly in the lumbar and thoracic spine, particularly in women after the menopause, though men are not exempt. People who are treated long term with steroids also are likely to develop osteoporosis. A sudden sharp pain is felt if a weakened vertebra collapses. Severe though this pain can be, it subsides with protective support and rest. The damaged bone heals, although it does not regain its original form.

Cancer deposits in the vertebral bodies can be a cause of deep seated and persistent pain in the lumbar and thoracic region, although not all deposits are painful. Some cancers produce firm dense deposits (prostate, breast) while others are more likely to erode and weaken bone causing collapse (lung). Radiotherapy to the spine can bring relief, although this is, of course, only part of the whole treatment of the underlying cancer.

The shoulder region

Much of the movement that we think of as shoulder movement really is made by the shoulder blade (scapula). Through the action of the powerful muscles which support it the scapula has a certain degree of freedom of movement up and down over the chest wall, carrying the shoulder joint with it (Figure 2.5). This mobility of the scapula is possible because its only bony connection with the rest of the skeleton is through the collar bone (clavicle). The outer end of the clavicle joins on to the strong bony spur which springs up from the back of the scapula, the acromion, in the acromio-clavicular joint. The acromion acts as a sturdy protective roof over the shoulder joint, so that when we carry a heavy load on our shoulder, or when a rugby forward pushes in the scrum the burden is borne by the scapula and the strain is taken by its supportive muscles. (Figure 2.6).

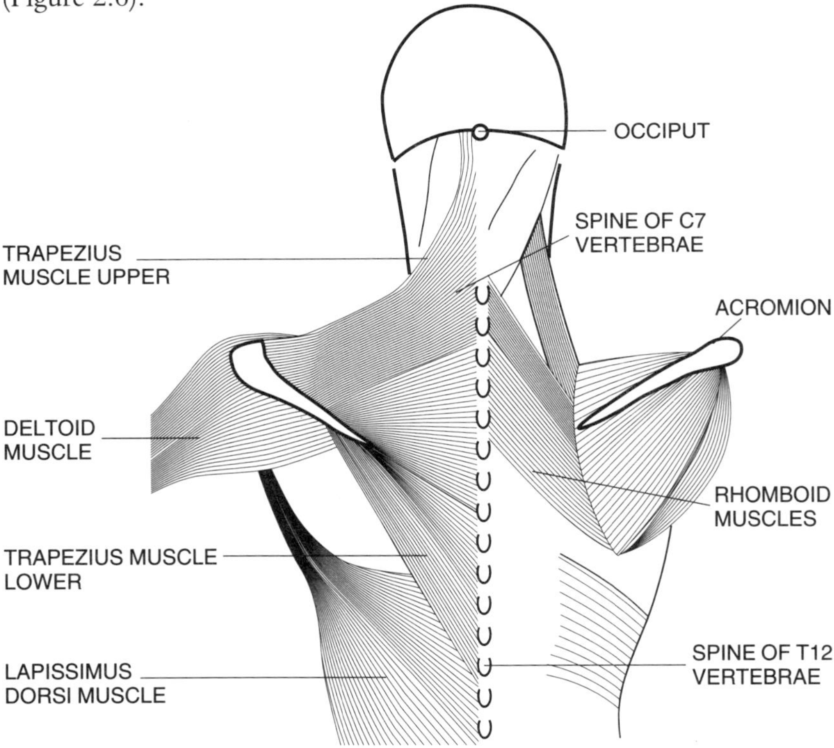

Figure 2.5: Muscles of the back – The trapezius muscle (left) runs from the back of the skull to the scapula and down the back. Beneath it (right) are other muscles which support the scapula.

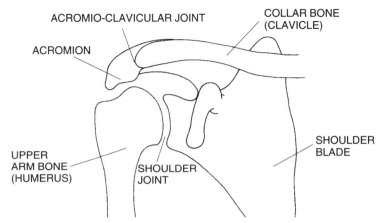

Figure 2.6: Shoulder joint – showing the bones which form the shoulder joint and the acromioclavicular joint

The shoulder girdle

This term refers to the scapula and clavicle and the muscles which support and control them, of which the most important is the trapezius muscle. The troubles that affect the shoulder girdle are therefore mainly muscular.

Muscle tension is chiefly felt in the upper part of the trapezius muscle and in the neighbouring neck muscles. Very often it is an unnecessary tension, reflecting our own emotional tension, perhaps due to anxiety, or to overeager attention, or just a bad postural habit. We can overcome this if we relax, and the painful spasm of the tense muscles is eased by warmth and massage which we can provide for ourselves. or ask for the help of an obliging friend.

Heavy loads carried by the arms pull downwards particularly on the upper section of the trapezius muscle and this is damaging if the muscle is not strong enough for its task. The downward drag may also harm the nerves which run downwards from the neck to the upper limb. For example, a young mother having to carry a heavy child may not only have aching shoulder girdle muscles but also an unpleasant form of neuralgia, giving her painful tinglings at night in the arm and hand. She may find relief from sleeping with the shoulder well supported by a pillow, or raising the whole arm. Strengthening exercise for the shoulder girdle muscles will help to prevent future trouble.

Referred pain from the neck can give rise to pain in the shoulder region and upper arm. The cause may lie in arthritis in the neck joints, irritating nerve roots and producing symptoms which are perceived as coming from the shoulder, arm or hand. Treatment should be directed to the neck and not to the shoulder or arm.

The shoulder joint

The shoulder joint is a ball and socket type of joint, but the socket is so shallow that it has to depend for stability on surrounding muscles and tendons. Closest to the joint is the "rotator cuff", which is a wrap-around group of small muscles springing from the front and the back of the scapula, running over the joint to be attached to the head of the upper arm bone, the humerus (Figure 2.7). Other supportive muscles include

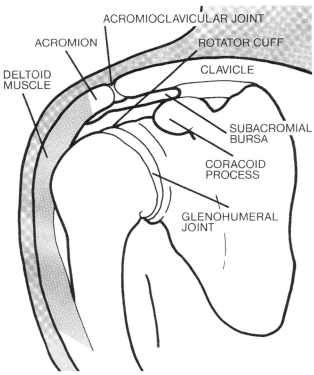

Figure 2.7: Shoulder joint – showing the rotator cuff and the subacromial bursa

the biceps and over all the powerful deltoid muscle, which moves the arm away from the body (abduction) and springs from the protective bony acromion above the shoulder.

Dislocation of the shoulder can happen nevertheless after a violent wrenching injury. The surgeon usually has little difficulty in reducing the dislocation but an anaesthetic is required to counter the painful spasm of the surrounding muscles.

A *rotator cuff tear* can follow a less serious wrenching injury. It is very painful and may cause blood to be shed into the shoulder joint. It requires rest and support with the arm in a sling, and gentle mobilisation as soon as pain permits.

Fracture through the head of the humerus is a common injury after a fall, requiring similar management – rest and support for the arm with a sling followed by a programme of exercises to regain mobility at the shoulder. Similar care is needed after any injury to the arm because of the effect it has in impairing shoulder movement.

Frozen shoulder is a state of persistent pain and immobility in the shoulder after any injury affecting the joint. It may also be the end result of a period of general immobility after a stroke or heart attack in which the arm is not used. Shoulder muscles, especially the deltoid, can waste rapidly and the joint itself can become restricted with fibrous adhesions. A long period of patient physiotherapy is needed with the patient encouraged to exercise shoulder movements.

Arthritis. Rheumatoid and similar forms of inflammatory arthritis commonly affect the shoulder. Pain and stiffness inhibit the use of the joint and muscles quickly waste, with the danger that a form of frozen shoulder may result. Pain relieving and anti–inflammatory drugs are needed as well as physical treatment, sometimes helped by an injection of cortisone. Arthritis can also affect the acromioclavicular joint, usually due to degenerative rather than inflammatory changes.

Subacromial bursitis. An important bursa lies between the top of the humerus and the overlying acromion: its purpose is to prevent friction between the two as the arm moves. Overuse of the shoulder may irritate the bursa, which becomes swollen and inflamed. Characteristically, this causes pain, not with the arm by the side, nor with the arm fully abducted at 90° but through an intermediate "painful arc" of about 30-60°. Resting the arm in a sling, with careful exercising will help. But to avoid the risk of shoulder stiffness, quicker relief can be given by an injection of cortisone into the bursa. It is not difficult for the doctor to do this painlessly using a local anaesthetic.

Our Feet

Our feet are wonderfully constructed. Each of them is prepared to bear our whole body weight on its padded sole and to accept the added stresses of walking, running and jumping. During our lifetime they walk hundreds of miles for us, moving in response to the powerful leg muscles as well as to the many small intrinsic foot muscles which move our toes. We owe our feet a debt of gratitude, but all too often we treat them with neglect. Sometimes we compress them into shoes in which appearances count for more than comfort.

The two arches of the foot are the secret of its success (Figure 2.8). The

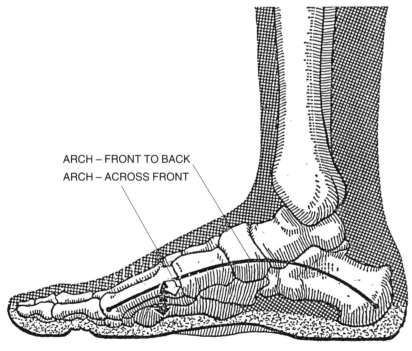

ARCH – FRONT TO BACK
ARCH – ACROSS FRONT

Figure 2.8: The foot arches – showing the longitudinal and the transverse arches

longitudinal arch runs from heel to toes, and the less obvious anterior (transverse) arch runs across the front of the foot, formed of the heads of the metatarsal bones, at the base of the toes. These arches are maintained not so much by the ligaments which hold neighbouring bones together as by the muscle power of the leg; the leg muscles send their tendons down into the feet, ending in attachments to the foot bones and to the toes. Their power helps to bind the interlocking foot bones together and to hold up the arches.

The height of the longitudinal arch varies in individuals. What may seem a flat arch in a child or young person is usually simply due to the natural flexibility of the foot at that age, changing to a more "normal" form as growth and strength progress. The anterior arch has the effect of putting the greater part of forefoot pressure on to the "ball" of the foot, i.e. the underside of the head of the metatarsal bone at the base of the big toe; less pressure is exerted beneath the head of the metatarsal of the little toe, and least of all beneath the intermediate toes. There is trouble if this arrangement fails.

Forefoot problems

Hallux valgus. In this common deformity the big toe is angled away from the midline, exposing the first metatarsal head to undue prominence and to the pressure of the shoe. A bunion may form over that prominence i.e. thickened skin, forming a callosity, sometimes with a bursa developing between the skin and the underlying bone (Figure 2.9). The usual cause of hallux valgus is a long period of badly fitting shoes which do not allow room for the big toe to lie straight. The chiropodist can apply a pad between the first and second toes, which helps matters, and care must then be taken to see that the shoe allows sufficient room without pressure.

Osteoarthritis often develops in the first big toe joint (metatarsophalangeal) secondary to hallux valgus, or it may develop while the toe is relatively straight (Hallux rigidus). In either case the joint is painful. If chiropody and shoe care cannot achieve comfort surgery may be needed. The orthopaedic surgeon removes a small portion of the first phalanx of the big toe, next to the joint. This allows the toe to lie straight and relieves pain. Prevention, of course, is the best answer. This means

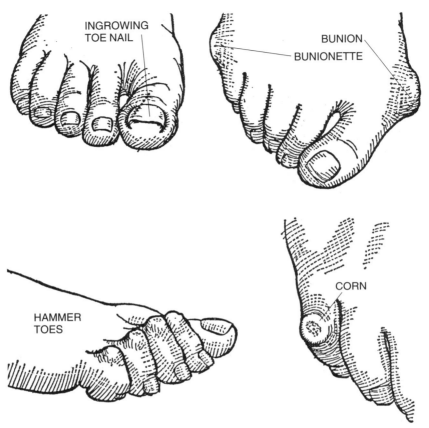

Figure 2.9: Common foot problems

two things: frequently going barefoot or shoeless indoors or (when safe) outdoors, and proper choice of shoe from childhood onwards. It is important to resist the temptation to let a growing child wear old shoes, instead of renewing them as soon as they begin to pinch.

Anterior arch failure. Weakened muscles and prolonged standing may lead to flattening of the anterior arch. This means that weight is borne in the wrong place, particularly by the heads of the second and third metatarsal bones. This is painful and to make things worse, a callus or corn forms on the sole of the foot beneath the displaced metatarsal head. An insole support will help: it is simple to make, cut from plastic material (ethyl vinyl acetate) and shaped to lie snugly in the shoe, it bears a central cushion-like pad. This is placed so as to lie just in front of the mid foot taking the weight off the tender metatarsal heads. In severe cases the answer may be an operation in which the surgeon removes the tip of the displaced metatarsal bone.

Rheumatoid arthritis is another cause of pain and tenderness in the forefoot. The arthritis can affect the joints at the base of the toes (metatarso–phalangeals) at an early stage, even beginning there, just as it may do in the corresponding joints in the hand (metacarpophalangeals).

Neuroma. A tender swelling occasionally forms on a nerve lying between the metatarsal bones in the forefoot. On standing, pressure on the forefoot compresses the nerve between the toes and is painful. A simple operation to remove the neuroma provides the cure.

Toe problems. Along with the forefoot troubles just described the small toes can develop painful deformities. The pull of their extensor tendons bends them up into the hammer toe position. Corns and calluses form on the angled top of the toes where they meet the pressure of the shoe (Figure 2.9). Toes may also become angled sideways so that they lie over or under each other. With their upward displacement, they pull on the protective padding tissue of the sole so that it no longer lies beneath the metatarsal heads as it should, adding to discomfort. Chiropody and careful padding with roomy shoes can do much to relieve discomfort. Specially moulded shoes can be made on a cast of the foot so that its shaped and padded sole follows the shape of the foot, distributing weight evenly. But if these measures are not enough the surgical operation of forefoot arthroplasty may be necessary. This means removing the tips of metatarsal bones which are causing pain, and also removing small portions of toe bones so that they may be straightened – in effect, redesigning the forefoot.

Circulatory disease. People with a poor foot circulation due to arteriosclerosis have an added risk of trouble. Pressure sores and minor injuries will take longer to heal, so that regular foot care is important.

Diabetes creates an even greater risk, for the person with diabetes has a tendency to arterial disease and also peripheral neuritis. This means that the sense of pain is dulled or lost so that the warning given by pain is absent, and pressure sores can develop unawares. Added to this, the extra sugar in the blood and tissues of a diabetic is helpful to any invading bacteria, and infection can develop more easily than in other people. The diabetic person must be taught to take extra foot care; a useful trick is to have a small mirror on the floor to make it easier to inspect the underside of the feet and toes every day.

Mid-foot problems

Fallen arch. As already mentioned, the appearance of a fallen arch in a child or young person generally proves to be unimportant and is corrected naturally as growth occurs and muscle strength increases. However, spastic flatfoot can be painful; it is due to an unusual bony formation in the mid foot, and will probably mean that a special support will have to be incorporated into the shoe. Rheumatoid and similar forms of arthritis cause mid-foot pain from failure of the longitudinal arch. An insole support is helpful, built up on its inner side, while general treatment for the arthritis will be directed towards combating the inflammation in the joints and strengthening muscle power.

High arch. A very high arch produces the foot deformity known as "pes cavus". It may result from contractures in the leg muscles after muscle disease such as myopathy. Forefoot problems are likely to develop as the body weight is thrown forwards on to the front of the foot.

Hind-foot problems

Plantar fasciitis. The plantar fascia is a layer of tough fibrous tissue within the sole of the foot; it is attached to the underside of the heel bone (calcaneus) at the back, and to the base of the toes at the front. Inflammation and pain may result from excessive stress on the sole of the foot through rough walking with inadequately protective shoes. It is also a feature of some kinds of arthritis, notably ankylosing spondylitis and Reiter's disease. (Chapters 5 and 6). Treatment is with rest, pain relieving and anti inflammatory drugs, gentle mobilisation of the feet, and, if necessary, soft insoles.

Calcaneal spur. A bony spur sometimes forms jutting forwards on the underside of the heel bone. It is the result of calcification in the hindmost fibres of the plantar fascia, and may be the after effect of plantar fasciitis. Pain can usually be relieved by a specially shaped supportive pad. taking the weight off the tender area. Radiation with ultrasound or diathermy may help, or a local injection of cortisone – carefully given, as the tissues in this area do not readily tolerate distension.

Ankle joint injury or arthritis can cause pain in the hind foot through its effect on the joints beneath the ankle bone (talus). Local heat and gentle mobilisation are needed, and shoes must give good support in the heel area.

Valgus heel. A fallen longitudinal arch and weakened leg muscles may result in the foot falling inwards and the heel bone becoming angled outwards (valgus); this commonly happens with advanced rheumatoid arthritis. To combat this displacement the inner side of the sole of the shoe is raised by a quarter of an inch or so, which allows the body weight to be borne more correctly.

3 | Osteoarthritis

Osteoarthritis is the commonest form of joint disease. It is second only to back pain in its call upon the GP's time. It is associated with age and it is estimated that 60% of people over 65 years of age have osteoarthritis in some form, although they are not necessarily aware of it. Osteoarthritis is essentially due to a wearing away of the all-important cartilage that covers the bone ends where they make contact in our joints – the articular cartilage.

Articular cartilage has some very special qualities. Its surface is smooth, pale and moist, and with the help of the small amount of fluid naturally present in the joint acting as a lubricant, the movement in a joint is virtually frictionless. Under the microscope it is seen that cartilage is composed of a network of connective tissue fibres (collagen) supporting the special cartilage component (proteoglycan) which gives it its strong resilient nature. This substance is formed by the cartilage cells which lie in the deeper layers near the junction of cartilage with bone. It can hold within it a certain amount of water and it is this which gives cartilage the ability to withstand considerable pressure without damage – something that is necessary in weight bearing joints.

The cause of osteoarthritis is usually explained as the combined effect of age plus wear and tear, though this is an oversimplification. Over the course of time the smooth surface of joint cartilage begins to fragment. Cartilage has only a limited capacity for repair and regrowth, so that its thickness becomes reduced, ultimately with irritation of the underlying bone. This is when pain begins. The effect on the partially exposed bone is to make it denser and also for it to form small bony outgrowths at the margin of the joint. These are called osteophytes and can be seen on an X-ray of the joint. The X-ray also shows a reduction in the gap between the two bones which form the joint, the gap revealing the reduced thickness of cartilage, which does not show on X-ray.

The joint capsule surrounds the joint (Figure 3.1) and is lined by a membrane, the synovial membrane (synovium), whose cells have a useful role. They are capable of absorbing and removing any debris shed into the joint cavity from damaged tissue. They are kept busy when the degenerative changes of osteoarthritis begin, so that the joint capsule becomes thickened due to its increased activity and this is a form of low grade inflammation. Hence the justification for the name *osteoarthritis*, implying inflammation as well as degeneration.

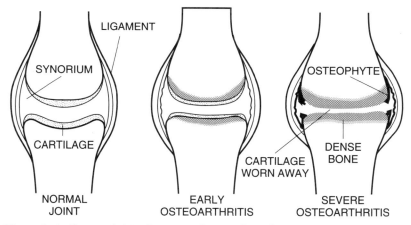

Figure 3.1: Osteoarthritis: Diagram showing how the articular cartilage is worn away and the underlying bone becomes denser

The stresses that may damage a joint include the extra load caused by a person being overweight, or years of excessive physical activity at work or in sport, or direct injury as with a fracture into or near a joint. A broken bone, if it unites imperfectly at an angle, can result in abnormal stress on a joint. Also the damage resulting from inflammatory arthritis such as rheumatoid arthritis can lead to the added development of osteoarthritis in the course of time.

Other factors. Certain other factors contributing to osteoarthritis are still not understood. Women are more susceptible to it than men, while some races are distinctly less affected than others. Heredity plays little part as a rule, although the node forming osteoarthritis of the hands tends to run in families, and there are some rare cases in which there is a strong family history of osteoarthritis developing at an early age. The features of osteoarthritis vary according to the joint affected as we shall see.

The symptoms can be summed up as "pain on use, stiffness after rest". In some situations pain may misleadingly be felt at a distance, as when hip disease gives rise to pain felt in the knee, or when there is pressure on a nerve as may happen in the neck.

The hand

The finger tip joints (distal interphalangeals) are the hand joints typically affected by osteoarthritis. In women the first signs may be at about the time of the menopause, and in men, who are less seriously affected, at a rather later age. At first there may be tenderness and swelling at one side or other of the joint, but this soon subsides and there is no further pain or tenderness. A small bony prominence, really an osteophyte, often forces the finger tip to one side making the finger crooked. These knobbly prominences are named Heberden's nodes after the physician who first described them some 200 years ago. A number of these nodes may form on the fingers of both hands (Figure 3.2). Although unsightly they cause very little trouble, are painless and interfere hardly at all with the use of the hand.

Base of thumb. Another joint often affected at the same time is the joint at the base of the thumb metacarpal where it joins the wrist. This can be painful when making any strong gripping movement with the thumb. On feeling over the joint line small osteophyte projections may be noted. If joint damage progresses, movement of the thumb away from the index finger (abduction) becomes restricted. Once the joint becomes painful we can spare it by making small changes in the way we use our hands e.g. by writing with a felt tipped pen, or pen and ink, rather than with a ball point pen which needs to be very firmly gripped. Or by not holding a heavy plate at a point near its rim, which requires a strong grip. Gentle

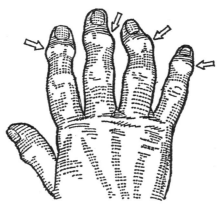

Figure 3.2: Heberden's nodes — These are small osteophytes which form at the margins of the finger tip joints

"round and round" movements of the thumb can be practised to maintain mobility, and firm massage around the base of the thumb, tending to pull the thumb away from the wrist.

Other joints in the hand are less seriously affected by osteoarthritis. The mid-finger joints (proximal interphalangeals) may suffer changes similar to those at the finger tip. Knobbly prominences here are called Bouchard's nodes. Sometimes one or more of the knuckle joints are affected (metacarpophalangeals). Pain and tenderness are not often severe, but if necessary can be eased by a warm hand bath and then massage to the hand and fingers, with a gentle pulling action tending to separate the bones of the affected joint.

Generalised osteoarthritis. When a number of hand joints are affected by osteoarthritis other, weight bearing joints may well become affected later, particularly the hip and knee. Such individuals have been found to have evidence of an inherited genetic predisposition to osteoarthritis.

The hip

Osteoarthritis of the hip is a major cause of pain and disability in older people. It affects more women than men and may begin at any age over fifty.

The normal hip is a perfectly functioning ball and socket joint. The head of the femur, covered with its smooth white cartilage looks like a shining billiard ball, fitting snugly into its socket similarly lined with cartilage. The shape of the hip joint gives it great stability, added to which it is surrounded on all sides by powerful muscles.

In some cases we can understand why things should begin to go wrong. The neck of the femur may have been fractured in a fall, and however carefully the surgeon may have repaired it with a well placed metal pin, the injury may have damaged the joint itself; perhaps even the necessary period of reduced mobility during healing harmed the joint. In childhood there is sometimes a fault in the growth and shaping of the neck and head of the femur, ultimately putting an abnormal strain on the hip joint. Excessive physical exercise at work or in sport, or being overweight may have started the trouble. But in many cases there is no obvious reason why the arthritis began and we can only speculate that there may have been some subtle fault in the structure of cartilage, or that there was some failure of blood supply to bone in the femoral head.

Symptoms. The first symptom is pain on standing or walking, and then stiffness after rest. Usually pain is felt in the hip and groin, spreading down into the thigh, although sometimes it seems to be only in the knee area. Examination soon shows that the knee is normal, but that hip movements are restricted. Swinging outwards (abduction) and rolling inwards (internal rotation) are limited. Pain becomes troublesome on walking, on going upstairs, or during the night.

Posture and gait are affected. The painful hip is more comfortable when held angled inwards towards the other leg (adduction). Unconsciously the patient adapts by tilting the pelvis upwards on the affected side, so as to make the two legs parallel. This has the effect of making the affected leg appear shorter and the other leg longer. Inevitably, the body weight comes to be borne more by the "longer" leg, so that the knee and the hip on that side suffer too. The patient begins to walk with a "dip" on the affected side, tending to hold the leg and foot turned outwards.

X-ray shows that the "joint space" (meaning the thickness of cartilage) in the affected hip is narrowed. Little osteophytes may have formed around the head of the femur, In advanced cases, the head of the femur may be misshapen and flattened i.e. worn away. But it must be said that the X-ray changes and the symptoms do not necessarily match: an alarming appearance on X-ray may not mean a very painful hip, and vice versa. (Figure 3.3)

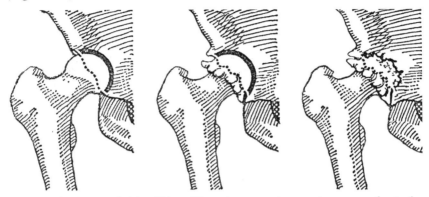

Figure 3.3: Osteoarthritis of hip – There is progressive wearing away of articular cartilage and formation of osteophytes

Treatment. The good news is that osteoarthritis of the hip does not inevitably progress. A limited amount of tissue healing can occur in the hip, and with helpful management this can be encouraged, mobility retained and progression halted or slowed down.

Exercise is important, ideally non weight bearing, and carried out "little and often". All movements – flexing and straightening, swinging the leg inwards and outwards, and rolling inwards and outwards should be encouraged. An initial period of instruction with a physiotherapist is important, including guidance on posture and walking, and the correct use of a walking stick should this be needed. If necessary, non weight bearing exercise can be given in the physiotherapy department with the weight of the leg borne by an overhead sling.

Hydrotherapy in a warm pool is helpful. It should begin under instruction in a therapy pool, and often can continue in a local swimming bath if there are sessions reserved for those with special needs, when the water can be made warmer.

Walking: As well as the use of a stick, a *raised sole* in the shoe on the affected side may be helpful as a raise of even a quarter of an inch helps compensate for the apparent leg shortening on that side.

Pain relief varies according to need. For mild pain there are a number of helpful herbal preparations. For more serious pain there is paracetamol, available for purchase over the counter. Some preparations combine it with codein, which has a constipating effect, or with aspirin, which can cause gastric irritation or bleeding, so care must be taken, particularly in the elderly. Ibuprofen is the safest of the non-steroidal anti inflammatory drugs, available without prescription as Nurofen.

Complementary therapies are discussed in Chapter 10.

Lifestyle. If hip pain has begun to affect daily activities adjustments will have to be made in the home. Loose mats and rugs must be removed for fear of tripping. A suitable chair is one with a firm, relatively high seat and side arms. The car seat may need adjustment or changing for better access. If high steps or stairs prove difficult, a wood block or tread may be interposed to halve the height of a step. As for *diet*, many claims are made of uncertain merit, and are more applicable to rheumatoid arthritis than to osteoarthritis. The usual medical advice is for a nutritious mixed diet, known to provide all necessary vitamins and minerals, especially calcium and vitamin D and to reduce weight where necessary. There is further discussion in Chapter 10.

Surgery. If pain and disability have reached the point of spoiling daily life the time has come to consider surgery. Hip replacement is one of the major surgical successes of the past 20 years. The secret of success lies in the cement which holds the artificial socket and femoral head firmly in place without any harm to the supporting bone (Figure 3.4). Nevertheless, it is a major operation, requiring the patient to be reasonably robust and to be prepared to face a period of rehabilitation afterwards. This will include retraining of muscles, and attention to posture and walking so as to overcome faults brought on by the arthritis.

Osteoarthritis can, of course affect both hips and if necessary the second damaged hip can be replaced, usually at an interval after the first. There are many people today who can testify to the success of bilateral hip replacement.

The Knee

The design of the knee makes it susceptible to injury in a number of ways. Excessive wear in use of the joint, combined with injury is the main reason for the eventual development of osteoarthritis.

The knee is basically a hinge joint, depending for its stability on strong ligaments on each side and within the joint, and on powerful muscles running from thigh to lower leg, particularly the quadriceps in front and the hamstrings behind. The thrust of weight bearing is borne by the two

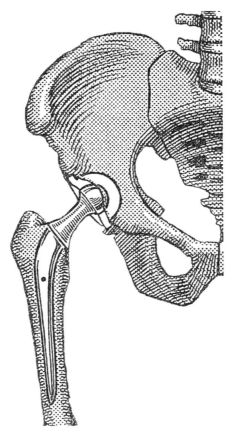

Figure 3.4: Hip replacement — The head of the metal prosthesis fits into the polyethylene socket and its shaft fits into the shaft of the femur

rounded condyles of the lower end of the femur, engaging with the flattened surface of the top of the tibia. On the top of the tibia sit the two semilunar cartilages (menisci), attached by their margins to the tibial head (Figure 3.5). Each cartilage is about a quarter of an inch thick at its outer

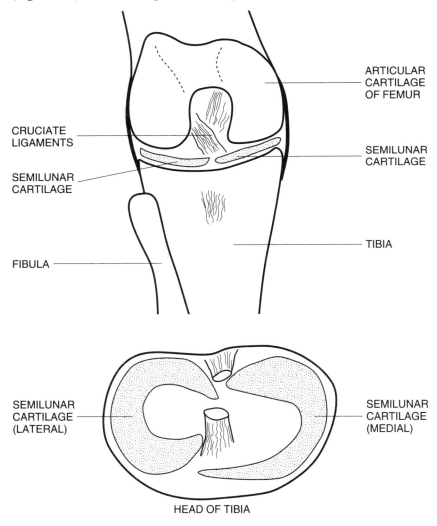

Figure 3.5: Knee anatomy – The bones of the right knee, without the patella (above) and the two semilunar cartilages on the head of the tibia (below)

edge, tapering off towards the centre, so helping to form a shallow hollow into which the condyle of the femur fits. In front of the knee is the patella, transmitting the pull of the quadriceps muscle in the front of the thigh down to the tibial head. The rear surface of the patella is covered with articular cartilage which is in contact with the cartilage over the condyles, sliding up and down as the knee bends and straightens.

Osteoarthritis can affect one part of the knee joint more than another, and often affects it all. In the contact surfaces of patella and femur, it causes pain and creakiness there, but its main effect is usually in the contact areas between femur and tibia, particularly in overweight people, and also in active people who have suffered the injury of a "torn internal cartilage". It is the medial semilunar cartilage which is most often damaged, usually by a violent twisting movement of the knee, common in footballers. A badly torn cartilage may have to be removed. This will be helpful in the short term but is liable to lead to osteoarthritis in later years.

Other events that may lead to osteoarthritis include fractures, of the patella or of the tibia, and any faulty alignment of the leg. "Bandy legs" (genu varus) for example means that the weight of the body is thrown mainly on to the inner part of the joint, and the opposite, "knock knee" (genu valgus) throws the weight on to the outer part of the joint. Another factor sometimes is the deposit of calcium crystalline substances within the tissue of the semilunar cartilages (chondrocalcinosis); these crystals may be released into the joint causing sudden severe pain, "pseudo gout" (Chapter 8).

Symptoms. *Pain* is the main symptom, on standing and walking, usually felt in both knees as both are likely to be affected. With movement there is a sense of creakiness *(crepitus)* which can be felt with a hand placed over the patella – and even heard.

Stiffness follows a period of rest and is worst on waking.

Swelling of the joint is due to accumulation of fluid, made more obvious if there is also thickening of the joint capsule. The swelling can be seen on either side of the patella and also for an inch or more above it, as the joint cavity is extensive.

Bleeding into the joint may follow injury, making the joint tensely swollen, hot and tender. Blood in any joint is slow to absorb and leaves a legacy of capsular thickening, fibrous adhesions within the joint which limit movement, and muscle wasting. It is important therefore that blood should be withdrawn from the joint as soon as possible.

Haemophilia. Bleeding into the knee can happen repeatedly after only minor injuries in boys and young men with haemophilia, often leaving badly damaged knees as a result. They need urgent treatment with the missing blood factor and withdrawal of blood from the joint as well as physical treatment to the knee.

Baker's cyst (popliteal cyst). The pressure of a persistent fluid effusion in the knee may force the joint membrane to form a cyst-like extension backwards, behind the knee. Fluid in the cyst may seal off or may remain in continuity with the knee joint. The cyst is not painful, but there is some danger that it may extend downwards, or leak fluid downwards into the calf muscles, which is painful. For this reason the cyst is best removed surgically.

Treatment. Much can be done at home to ease the pain of an osteo-arthritic knee and to strengthen the leg muscles. A hot compress is the simplest, made from a small towel soaked in hot water, wrung out and wrapped round the knee for some minutes. A plastic or waterproof layer should be put between the skin and the compress. After removal of the hot compress the joint is massaged with oil or liniment and exercised.

Isometric exercises cannot be performed too often as the strength of the thigh muscle helps to stabilise and protect the knee. This means resting the leg straight on a couch and then rhythmically tensing and relaxing the thigh muscles – tightening the muscles but not moving the joint.

Physiotherapy. In the physiotherapy department various forms of electrotherapy are available – infrared radiation, shortwave diathermy, ultrasound therapy and microwave therapy. usually given at the physiotherapists discretion, with instruction in appropriate exercises. This might include sitting on the side of a couch with the knee at 90 degrees and regularly straightening the knees, perhaps with a weight added around the ankle to build up quadriceps power.

Hydrotherapy is valuable in allowing similar exercises and movements to be carried out in a weight free environment, under instruction.

Walking exercises help to improve gait and confidence. If necessary, weight bearing can be assisted so as to lessen the strain on the knees by using parallel bars to give hand holds on each side, Axillary or elbow crutches can also be used if necessary.

Taping the patella. If knee pain is mainly arising from friction between the patella and the femur, the simple application of broad adhesive tape over the front of the patella round to the inner side of the knee can help; it does this by pulling the painful surfaces slightly apart. This eases the pain of friction and also, after some days, may allow some degree of healing of the damaged cartilage surfaces. In some cases the tape may have to run from the patella to the outer side of the knee to separate the inner part of the patella from the femur.

Aspiration and injection. A persistent effusion of fluid in the knee joint is best removed by needling under local anaesthetic. This is not difficult and can be carried out in the GP's surgery or in the hospital clinic. It does require scrupulous attention to an aseptic technique in order to avoid infection. After withdrawal of fluid an injection of steroid (cortisone) is often given, bringing rapid relief of symptoms which may last for weeks or months. However, such injections should not be given too often: the relief of pain may be too much of a good thing, and encourage the patient to use the knee excessively.

Irrigation. If the joint fluid is found to be thickened with debris from tissue damage, the withdrawal of fluid may be followed by irrigation – washing out the joint cavity with saline. This too helps relieve pain

Arthroscopy is the technique for examining the interior of a joint by internal inspection through a tiny telescope inserted under local anaesthetic. The knee is the joint that is best suited to this form of examination. The operator can inspect the state of the joint cartilage and the joint lining, and can see whether the semilunar cartilage has been damaged. If necessary a small amount of tissue can be removed for examination under the microscope. Irrigation of the knee is a normal preliminary to arthroscopy, so as to fill the joint with clear fluid in order for the operator to see. This means that arthroscopy and the irrigation that goes with it are a form of treatment as well as being useful in diagnosis.

Drugs and lifestyle. Here the recommendations are the same as those made for the care of the osteoarthritic hip (above).

Surgery. With osteoarthritis of the knee as with the hip, joint damage may progress to the point where pain is seriously limiting daily living, and treatment has not brought relief. Can surgery help? *Knee replacement* surgery has developed greatly in the past 20 years. A number of different designs (prostheses) have evolved for replacing the knee, based on a combination of metal and polyethylene plastic. As with the hip, success depends on the cement firmly holding the prosthesis in place in the bone of femur and tibia, on the quality of the bone (fortunately usually good in an osteoarthritic joint), on the skill and experience of the surgeon, and last but not least, on the work and co-operation of the patient. Considerable determination is required from the patient in working for success, both in preparation for the operation and afterwards during rehabilitation. The knee depends for its stability so much on muscle power that this aspect of post operative care is even more important after knee surgery than it is after hip replacement.

Other operations are sometimes indicated. *Removal* of the patella is helpful if the bone has been fractured or if its cartilage surface is badly eroded while the rest of the knee is little affected. The knee joint can still work surprisingly well without a patella. *Osteotomy* is an operation which cuts through the lower femur or upper tibia and reunites the bone at a better angle when this has previously been faulty. It helps to relieve joint pain.

Osteoarthritis of spine

Osteoarthritis affects two regions of the spine in particular, lumbar and cervical, the lumbar region because it is subjected to the heaviest loads, and the cervical because it is the most mobile part of the spine. The name given to spinal osteoarthritis is *spondylosis,* implying that it is primarily a degenerative process. This should not be confused with *spondylitis,* which refers to an inflammatory process in the spine, as with ankylosing spondylitis, which is described in Chapter 6.

Lumbar spondylosis

The cause. Lumbar spondylosis is generally thought to be the result of long years of hard physical work, lifting and moving heavy loads. possibly incurring disc prolapses as well. Damp too is popularly supposed to play a part, but there is no proof of this, for spondylosis can develop in a dry climate as well as in a damp one. Older women may develop spondylosis too, meaning that the strains of domestic work may be enough to affect the spine. Also, the repeated small jolting shocks transmitted upwards from heel to spine in walking on hard surfaces may play a part.

There is a general reduction in the height of the intervertebral discs as they degenerate, and this brings into contact the rounded margins of the vertebral bodies. The resulting irritation of the bony surfaces causes the outgrowth of osteophytes. Sometimes these are big enough to make contacts like bony bridges between neighbouring vertebrae (Figure 3.6). In addition there is degeneration of cartilage in the pairs of small joints (facetal joints) at the back of each vertebra that articulate with the pair above and the pair below.

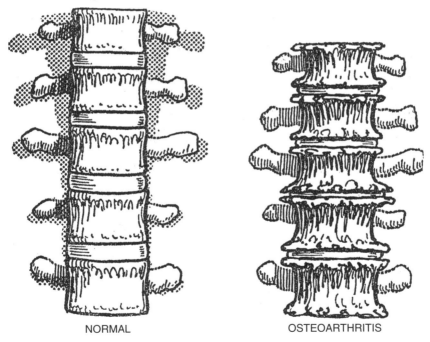

NORMAL   OSTEOARTHRITIS

Figure 3.6: Osteoarthritis of lumbar spine – The intervertebral discs have worn thin and osteophytes have formed at the margins of the vertebrae

Symptoms. The *pain* of lumbar spondylosis is of a deep gnawing nature within the lower back spreading to some extent to the waist and hips. It is made worse by movement, and also by sitting or lying in a bad position, and improved if the back is held straight in a chair with a firm lumbar support or on a firm mattress. *Stiffness* can be severe especially after sitting or lying in a bad position, and is largely due to protective spasm in the muscles of the lower back. *Rigidity* of the lower back is the result of the reduction in spinal movement. *Nerve root pressure* may result if osteophytes and other changes in the spine press on spinal nerves as they emerge from the spine; this will be perceived as pain in the thigh or lower leg.

Treatment. Simple care at home can bring much relief.

Warmth eases pain and muscle spasm, most simply given with a hot bottle or infrared lamp. Warm clothing too is important, protecting from cold and draughts.

Massage relieves spasm, given with the sufferer lying face downwards, using warm oil or liniment, applied with a firm hand. *Posture* is always important, the aim being to keep the spine straight, whether standing, sitting or lying, paying attention to lumbar support in armchair and car seat, and having a firm internally sprung mattress on the bed. If necessary this can be reinforced by a light weight board under the mattress.

The Alexander method teaches an awareness of posture and of movement, which is valuable for back sufferers.

Exercise must be of a gentle nature, with spinal bending and turning as much as pain will allow, and performed "little and often". A short daily walk is important, but not over hard or rough ground; shoes should have soft soles that absorb shocks. Trainers are useful here. A walking stick is helpful for support and stability.

Physiotherapy. Short wave diathermy or ultrasonic radiation given at the physiotherapist's discretion, helps by penetrating the back more than simple surface warmth can. The therapist can also advise over problems of posture and exercise

Hydrotherapy in a warm pool allows exercise to be undertaken more freely, and an added refinement in some pools is the presence of hot underwater jets set in the pool wall at convenient heights to play on the lower back and other areas, such as shoulder, neck and knee.

Drugs. Pain relieving drugs are very likely to be needed. The policy should be to keep their use to an acceptable minimum, omitting them whenever possible to avoid habituation. The range of drugs available is similar to that described under osteoarthritis of the hip and there is further comment in Chapter 10.

TENS stimulator. This equipment gives small electrical stimuli through two electrodes which adhere to the skin; the strength of the stimuli can be varied. This has an effect like that of acupuncture, of blocking out the sensation of pain. For relief of low back pain the electrodes are placed on either side of the midline on the back in the painful area. The user maintains the stimulus for several minutes according to need. This simple piece of equipment has the advantage of providing safe use at home and helping to reduce the need for pain relieving drugs.

Spinal corset. A light weight corset has a place if pain is anticipated during a period of activity or travel; it is better if at all possible not to rely on a corset for permanent support.

Surgery does not usually have a role in the management of lumbar spondylosis, unless there is some other feature in its favour. Sometimes instability develops between a pair of lumbar vertebrae. in which case spinal fusion with a bone graft is indicated.

Depression. Any persistent pain for which there is no ready relief is likely to cause depression, or to enhance any tendency to depression already present. A change of regime, introduction of a TENS stimulator, a period at a spa specialising in rheumatic treatment – any of these will help combat depression and if necessary, a period of treatment with an anti depressive drug will help.

Cervical spondylosis

Degeneration in the intervertebral discs begins at a rather earlier age in the neck than in the lower back. Undoubtedly this is due to the mobility of the cervical spine rather than to weight bearing (except in countries where heavy loads are habitually carried on the head). Around the margins of the discs, as they degenerate, pressure is applied on underlying bone, leading to the outgrowth of irregular bony osteophytes. There is a danger that these may encroach on the spaces through which the spinal nerves emerge giving rise to pain and numbness (Figure 3.7). Also the cartilage of the small facetal joints may deteriorate causing pain and local muscle spasm.

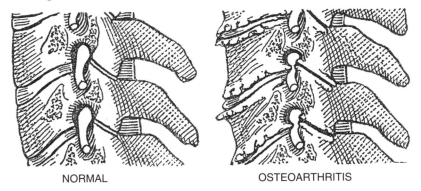

NORMAL   OSTEOARTHRITIS

Figure 3.7: Osteoarthritis of cervical spine – Here the osteophytes can compress the emerging nerve roots

Neck injuries may aggravate these changes. A *whiplash* injury in a head-on car crash flings the head violently forwards, after which it rebounds back, wrenching ligaments between vertebrae and damaging the discs. *Dislocation* is the worst form of neck injury, as from diving head first into a shallow pool. Here the greatest danger is of damage to the spinal cord, causing permanent paralysis in the lower limbs.

Symptoms. Cervical spondylosis causes pain in the neck and also in the surrounding neck muscles which are tender with protective spasm. There is stiffness and restriction of neck movement, especially on sideways flexion (ear to shoulder movement). Most people over 40 are aware of creakiness and probably discomfort on bending and twisting the neck. The most affected area is of the 4th, 5th and 6th vertebrae, where neck movement is normally greatest. Pressure on an emerging nerve root at this level gives rise to numbness and tingling in the shoulder and arm.

Treatment. Simple and effective home treatment is readily available. *Warmth* can be applied by hot bottle, electric pad or infrared lamp. *Massage* follows, self administered or from a helper, firmly and gently working on the neck muscles, going down to the trapezius muscle of the shoulder girdle. *Aromatherapy:* essential oil such as lavender may used for this, or a liniment with less attractive fragrance. *Traction* is helpful, most simply given by hand during massage; a more elaborate form is given with a light harness under the jaw, connected by a cord to a pulley and weight of 2lbs or more, which can be applied for longer periods.

A *collar* is protective against the pain of any slight movement. An inflatable collar supporting the back of the neck is a convenient aid when travelling. For longer use a sorbo collar can be worn; it should be trimmed carefully for size and worn in a stockinette sheath. If a very firm collar is needed after neck injury one can be made of plastic, if necessary with a metal frame: this type should be fitted by a specialist in such equipment (podiatrist).

TENS stimulator. For relief of chronic severe pain this equipment is valuable and convenient for home use (see under lumbar spondylosis).

Drugs for pain relief should only be taken according to need so as to avoid habituation. The simplest are herbal remedies, after which there is paracetamol, sometimes combined with other agents such as dextropropoxyphene (co-proxamol) or aspirin or codein. With long standing cervical spondylosis in which there may be an element of inflammation, one of the non-steroidal anti inflammatory (NSAID) drugs is justified of which ibuprofen is the safest, available without prescription as Nurofen.

4 | Rheumatoid arthritis

Rheumatoid arthritis is an inflammatory disease of joints which can, in time, have a damaging effect on mobility and health. It is estimated that it affects over a million people in the UK, three quarters of whom are women. It begins most often in middle adult life from 30 to 60 years of age, but literally no age is exempt, from childhood to old age. It varies very much in its severity and in the fluctuations in its course. In its mildest forms it may subside leaving little or no lasting damage; if more severe it causes some degree of disability. It may undermine general health and can lead to complications affecting other parts of the body such as the eyes, nerves and lungs. Research has taught us much about the nature and mechanisms of the inflammation it causes, and we know it to be an auto immune disease, but its fundamental origin is still not fully understood.

Immune system. We are all familiar with the immune system as the source of antibodies which circulate in the blood in our defence ready to combat or neutralise invading germs and their toxins. It also has another function, the provision of *cellular immunity*. This is based on the action of white cells, lymphocytes, which are primed to recognise and attack foreign or abnormal cells which could harm us. They have the ability to distinguish between normal body cells ("self") and abnormal cells (identified as "not self") against which they set up an inflammatory reaction. This is the "rejection reaction" that has to be avoided or suppressed if a surgical transplant is to succeed.

In rheumatoid arthritis a change occurs in cells that line the joint membrane (synovial cells) so that they become identified as "not self" and come under attack. As a result, large numbers of lymphocytes and other cells migrate into the joint lining and start up inflammation (synovitis) producing the four classical symptoms of inflammation: heat, redness, swelling and pain.

To some extent, people who develop rheumatoid arthritis are predisposed to it, for the majority carry identifiable tissue cell "markers". One effect of the inflammation is to produce antibodies, among which is the *rheumatoid factor* whose presence in the blood helps to confirm the diagnosis. If present in high levels, the rheumatoid factor gives us a warning that the arthritis might become severe and affect organs other than the joints. People with a positive blood test for rheumatoid factor are said to be "seropositive"; absence of the factor usually means that the arthritis is milder ("seronegative").

Symptoms. The main symptoms of rheumatoid arthritis are pain, swelling and stiffness in the affected joints. It most often begins in the knuckles (metacarpophalangeals) of the hands or the corresponding joints in the feet. Sometimes it will develop quickly, almost overnight, and in other cases much more gradually, over a matter of weeks. It can spread to other joints: the wrists, ankles, elbows, knees, shoulders, hips and neck, though usually only some of these are involved. Its pattern of distribution is noticeably symmetrical i.e. affecting the same joints on both sides of the body. Unlike osteoarthritis, it does not affect the joints of the fingertips, although it can affect the midfinger joints. Morning stiffness is a striking feature, and can last for an hour or more.

Continuing joint inflammation is harmful to general health and well-being, and explains the sense of fatigue and lack of energy which trouble many people with rheumatoid arthritis. There is usually anaemia, too, due to the depressive effect of the arthritis on the bone marrow; if this is at all marked it will add to the sense of fatigue and also cause breathlessness.

Joint damage. Inflammation in an affected joint causes thickening of the joint lining and distension of the joint with fluid. The process is most active in the recess where the joint lining is attached around the end of the bone near its covering of cartilage. In the course of time inflammation erodes the cartilage and even the underlying bone, and weakens the ligaments which hold the two bone ends in close contact (Figure 4.1). In the hand, the pull of the tendons, acting on the damaged knuckles, draws the fingers over to the little finger side (Figure 4.2) producing the

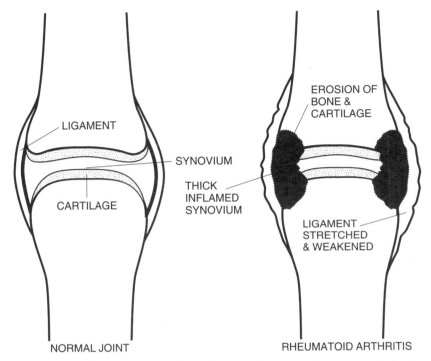

Figure 4.1: Rheumatoid Arthritis – Diagram showing inflammatory thickening of synovium with erosion of cartilage and bone

characteristic hand appearance of rheumatoid arthritis.

If the inflammation is not checked by treatment the end result can be a badly damaged joint, its eroded cartilage causing pain and limiting movement, the weakened ligaments making the joint unstable and disuse making neighbouring muscles weak and wasted. If an inflamed joint is rested for long periods in a bent position there is danger of it developing a *flexion deformity* e.g. a knee so affected could not be straightened, perhaps by a matter of 20 or 30 degrees. This is very difficult to overcome, but should be prevented with proper care.

Local complications. Fibrous *nodules* beneath the skin at pressure points are one of the features of rheumatoid arthritis; they often appear over the ulna bone near the point of the elbow. Nodules may form at many other sites, such as in the finger *tendons* and their *tendon sheaths* causing trigger finger or tendon rupture. *Bursitis* is common too, either at a pressure point or near a joint. Swelling of the wrist joint can be responsible for *carpal tunnel syndrome* (Chapter 2). Bones too suffer from the presence of inflammation in neighbouring joints and from disuse producing *osteoporosis*.

Distant complications in other body systems can develop in later years with seropositive rheumatoid arthritis. The underlying cause is a form of inflammation in small blood vessels, *vasculitis*. In the *fingers* this interferes with the circulation causing cold fingers. Many people with rheumatoid arthritis have *dry eyes* as a result of failure of the tear glands, also *episcleritis* which produces a reddened patch on the white of the eye; it is painless

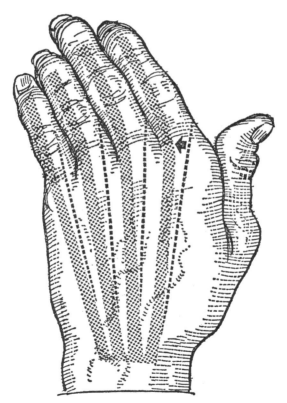

Figure 4.2: The hand in RA – The effect of the arthritis is to allow tendons to pull the fingers over to the little finger side (ulnar deviation)

and quickly subsides. The *nerves* can be affected by peripheral neuritis which can cause a mild numbness of the feet and hands, or sometimes can affect a single nerve such as one in the leg which causes weakness in the muscles which raise the foot. In the *lungs* there may be nodule formation, and fibrosis or *pleurisy* with a collection of fluid, but in time this subsides. Inflammation of the surface of the *heart* is quite common (pericarditis); usually it is mild, does not impair the heart's action and often goes unnoticed, subsiding naturally. Very occasionally the heart valves can be affected.

Course and outlook. All of this may seem alarming but it must be remembered that only a small proportion of people with rheumatoid arthritis become badly affected. Table 3 shows that only 5% develop the most disabling kind of arthritis with complications. In other words, of 20 people, on average, who have had rheumatoid arthritis for 20 years 4 will remain unaffected in their activities, 4 will be left with only minor trouble, 7 will have appreciable difficulties, 4 will have more serious problems, and only one will be unfortunate enough to progress to bad disability. So if your doctor tells you that you have rheumatoid arthritis it is quite wrong to start thinking "When do I order my wheel chair?" There is a great deal that treatment can offer. And you must remember that a doctor's impression is all too often formed from the more serious patients who return frequently to him for help, and he tends to forget about those who have done well and never need to come back to him.

Twenty years after developing rheumatoid arthritis the condition of 20 patients will be as follows:

4 will have recovered fully	20%
4 will have minor trouble only	20%
7 will have appreciable trouble	35%
4 will have quite serious trouble	20%
1 will be badly disabled	5%
20	100%

Table 3: Rheumatoid arthritis: the outcome after 20 years

Stress. For rheumatoid arthritis as with any long lasting disorder, stress will make things worse, so that relief from stress is an important part of patient care. For the young housewife the stresses of providing everyday care for children and household make it all the more difficult to cope with the discomforts of painful joints. For the working man there is the anxiety of continuing his daily job and travel in spite of the arthritis, trying not to lose time from work. For the older woman a flare-up in the arthritis may coincide with some crisis such as a divorce or a bereavement in the family. Joyful occasions too can make their demands: "My daughter is getting married next month and I MUST be on my feet for the reception!".

Treatment

The treatment of rheumatoid arthritis begins with self care at home. This requires an understanding of the care that must be taken of painful joints and of health in general. When further help is needed it is given by a medical team in which the GP is backed up by the resources of a hospital clinic. Here specialist doctors and expert therapists, provide treatment, aids and other help and sometimes surgery. Complementary medicine too has its place. In all, it should be a holistic approach, caring for all aspects of a patient's needs.

Home care

Rest is necessary for an inflamed joint, with support from a splint or sling as appropriate. The joint should be held in a position which is comfortable but at the same time avoiding a position which would be undesirable should the joint stiffen. For the wrist this would mean holding it slightly bent upwards (extended); for the knee the best position should be straight or only very slightly bent (flexed). When resting the leg on a bed or couch it might seem kind to place a pillow under the knee but this is wrong because, were it to stiffen, say, flexed at an angle of 40 degrees this would be most undesirable.

Movement. A rested joint should be moved frequently through as full a range as pain permits. If pain is severe, the movement must obviously be gentle and passive i.e. carried out by a helper. But if at all possible, joints should be moved by normal muscle power so as to keep the muscles in use and avoid muscle wasting. Unaffected joints should be moved and exercised too for the same reason.

Compresses. A cold compress will help to cool a inflamed joint. A hot compress should not be used, although it may help when inflammation has subsided, as in the treatment of an osteoarthritic joint.

Infrared radiation from a lamp is helpful over shoulders, neck and knees, but should not be used over an acutely inflamed joint. Otherwise it is helpful in combination with simple massage and exercise at home e.g. for the shoulders making sure that full abduction is achieved (raising the arms sideways to 90 degrees) and full rotation (touching the back of the head with the finger tips, and touching the middle of the back)

Massage may be given, not over or near an inflamed joint, but over adjoining muscles, which can also be given gentle isometric tensing exercises, especially in the case of the quadriceps in the thigh, as described in the care of osteoarthritis of the knee.

Rest for the whole person is necessary when the arthritis is in an active phase and causing fatigue. This may be difficult to arrange, but quiet rest periods of as little as 15 or 20 minutes are worth while two or three times a day. At night a relaxing hot bath is an important aid to the night's sleep. In the morning simple limb massage and general exercises help to dispel the morning stiffness characteristic of rheumatoid arthritis.

Hand baths help to relieve stiff and painful hand and finger joints. They are most simply given by immersing the hands in a bowl of comfortably hot water while wearing a pair of light weight plastic gloves to protect the skin. After a few minutes immersion the gloves are removed, the hands dusted with talcum powder and a few more minutes are spent in hand and finger exercise. Particular care should be given to keeping the fingers straight, as in the prayer position, so as to avoid any tendency for finger joints to become fixed in a flexed position.

Physiotherapy

This usually means attending a hospital department for physical therapies that cannot readily be undertaken at home – much as described in Chapter 3 but with certain differences.

Exercises are given under supervision for all affected joints, with special attention to shoulders, hips and knees. Often the weight of the affected limb is supported in a sling to assist movement. The aim is to improve the range of movement of a joint where this has been reduced, and to build up strength in weakened muscles.

Walking exercises are given, if necessary with the aid of parallel bars or a mobile walking aid (Zimmer type) for those with severe lower limb problems. This gives an opportunity to assess the need for a raised sole in one or other shoe, or to practice walking up steps.

Radiation. Infrared or ultrasonic radiation can be given to the region of a joint, possibly combined with massage, prior to exercise

Wax baths are helpful for affected hands. Wax with a specially low melting point is heated in a small bath, into which the hands are repeatedly dipped until they are coated like a glove with a layer of hot wax. After some minutes this is peeled off and the hands and fingers are exercised.

Faradic foot baths are sometimes used to give electrical stimulation to foot muscles in order to increase their power

Splints. Special removable splints can be made with fibreglass or plaster of Paris to rest and support the lower leg when there is knee arthritis, or for the wrist and hand. If the therapist is working on a knee with a flexion deformity in order to try and straighten it, a series of rest plasters can be made at intervals as the joint gradually becomes straighter.

Neck treatments must be given with great care when exercising; rheumatoid arthritis can produce instability in the neck joints so that vigorous movements must be avoided for fear of dislocation.

A neck *collar* of sorbo rubber or a firmer one of plastic is a valuable support, but must be properly fitted.

Hydrotherapy. Personally supervised exercise in a warm pool is very helpful for shoulder, hip and knee movement. It is tiring for the patient and should not continue for more than 20 minutes; it should be followed by a rest period with the patient wrapped in a warm towel.

Complementary therapies. *Acupuncture* can be helpful in the relief of pain, so reducing the need for pain relieving drugs. The *Alexander method* is also valuable in helping to maintain a good posture and well co-ordinated movement. For further comments on diet see Chapter 10.

Occupational therapy

The most valuable task of the occupational therapist is the careful assessment of the needs of the patient with arthritis. For women patients in particular this means judging what help they need in carrying out everyday household tasks – in dressing, washing, preparing food in the kitchen, operating taps, doorknobs etc. A large array of useful aids are available (see Appendix).

Social worker. The social worker can advise on services that are available from the local authority such as home helps, bath attendants and mobility allowance.

Drug treatment

Drugs of different types play an important part in the treatment of rheumatoid arthritis, but some of them are powerful and their use must be monitored with care.

Analgesics are pure pain relievers and do not have any action against inflammation. *Paracetamol* is an example, and so is its combination with dextropropoxyphene and with codein.

Combined analgesic and anti inflammatory drugs are much used. This includes some herbal preparations, *aspirin* on its own and in combination .But aspirin can damage the stomach and cause bleeding and so, if taken, is safer in an enteric coated form.

Non steroid anti inflammatory drugs (NSAIDs) are quite powerful and effective, but some may irritate the stomach. *Ibuprofen* is the safest and is available without prescription as Nurofen. All the others are best given under medical supervision.

"Disease modifying drugs" acting over a period reduce the inflammation of rheumatoid arthritis; they should only be given under medical supervision with some form of monitoring. *Sulphasalazine* is the safest. The anti malarial drugs *Chloroquin* and *Hydroxychloroquin* are gently acting, but require specialist eye checks periodically, although in fact they rarely affect the eyes. *Gold injections* (Myocrysin) and tablets (Auranofin) are both effective in the long term, but can have serious side effects on the skin, blood and kidneys. The same applies to *Penicillamine*.

Immunosuppressive drugs such as *Methotrexate* are only used in the most serious cases and require close monitoring.

Steroids

Steroid drugs, meaning cortisone and its derivatives such as prednisone have a rapid and powerful effect in checking inflammation in rheumatoid arthritis, whether given by mouth (systemically) or by injection into a joint. But their excessive use when first introduced led to serious side effects: fragile skin, bruising and bleeding, stomach ulcers and osteoporosis. Consequently systemic steroids came to be avoided or only given as a last resort when joint damage was already advanced. The current tendency is to use modest doses (e.g. prednisone 5 or 7.5 mg daily) given early in the course of arthritis if this is seen to be actively progressing. The daily dose is kept low or reduced with the help of other drugs as "steroid sparers".

Local injections are widely used, especially for swollen painful knees. Under a local anaesthetic as much joint fluid as possible is withdrawn with syringe and needle and then a small volume of long lasting steroid is injected. Relief is rapid (patients in one American clinic clamour for "another shot of joy juice, doc!") Movement and exercises to build up muscle power can begin again. However, these injections must not be given too often or the joint will be damaged by overuse. An average frequency limit for a individual joint is probably 4 times a year. Other sites often helped by steroid injections are the shoulder, tendon sheaths, carpal tunnel, and finger joints.

Surgery

As described under osteoarthritis, surgical replacement of a hip or knee when damaged beyond repair can give great relief. But the situation is not quite so favourable with rheumatoid arthritis, for the quality of bone is impaired by osteoporosis in the neighbourhood of an inflamed joint, coupled with the effect on muscles of relative disuse. This means that the surgeon must take great care with his technique, also that preparation for the operation and post operative care must be intensive. Other joint replacements have been developed for the shoulder, elbow, ankle and finger joints.

5 | Other forms of arthritis

There are other forms of arthritis which superficially resemble rheumatoid arthritis, but they differ in their causes and in the end result. They are "seronegative", lacking the rheumatoid factor. Among other things this means that the nodule formation, so characteristic of rheumatoid arthritis, is absent and the pattern of joint involvement is different. These other forms of arthritis have important links with the skin, bowel, eyes and spine and some have a known infective cause. Arthritis in children, too, differs from arthritis in adults and is included here.

Psoriatic arthritis

Psoriasis is a common skin disease. It appears as roughly circular patches of reddened scaly skin, which peel and flake readily but do not itch. These patches form often over the knees and elbows but can appear anywhere. If the scalp is involved there is much shedding of scurf, like dandruff. The finger and toe nails may be affected too, with tiny pitted marks and a heaping up of tissue beneath the nail. Psoriasis may develop at any age. It affects both sexes and is often familial. It has a variable course and tends to improve in summer weather when the skin is exposed to sunlight.

Arthritis develops in up to 10% of people with psoriasis. In those who have psoriasis of the nails, the arthritis mainly affects the finger tip joints and the corresponding joints in the toes. These joints become swollen and tender, and sometimes the whole of a finger or toe swells with a sausage like appearance. After rest and treatment the inflammation subsides, but sometimes with loss of bone, leaving a shortened lax finger.

In other individuals the arthritis affects the knee, ankle, elbow or wrist in no particular order. In yet others, arthritis begins at the base of the spine in the sacro-iliac joints and spreads upwards in a pattern identical with ankylosing spondylitis. These usually are people who have inherited the HLA–B27 cell marker as spondylitic patients do.

The *end result* of psoriatic arthritis is in most cases less damaging than in rheumatoid arthritis, except for those who suffer a lot of erosion of bone ends in the fingers. With spinal involvement, the result is just as it is in ankylosing spondylitis – a stiffened back or neck, but painless and, if properly cared for, in good position with very little disability.

Treatment of the *skin* in psoriasis helps the arthritis too. The conventional medical treatment is with ointments and lotions derived from coal tar, including dithranol and also salicylic acid, which have the effect of loosening the thick scales of skin. For the scalp, preparations are available for use as shampoos. In milder forms, herbal preparations are helpful such as Aloe vera and Evening primrose.

Treatment of the *arthritis* is very similar to that of rheumatoid arthritis. During a period of active arthritis an affected joint must be rested and protected with splint or sling and pain relieving or NSAID drugs given as necessary. As inflammation subsides, the joint must be carefully mobilised with exercises for limb muscles as described under physiotherapy for rheumatoid arthritis. If the psoriasis and the arthritis are both severe an immunosuppressive drug can be used: azathioprine and methotrexate act against both the skin and the joint conditions, but they are powerful drugs that should only be given under close medical supervision.

Reiter's disease

In Reiter's disease there are three main symptoms: arthritis, conjunctivitis and urethritis (inflammation of the urethra with pain on passing water). These all develop within two or three weeks of either a sexually acquired urethritis or an acute bowel infection such as dysentery. The acquired urethritis resembles gonorrhoea, but that is not necessarily the cause, for it may be due to a virus or other organism. When Reiter's disease follows dysentery urethritis is part of the disease and does not have a sexual origin. Reiter's disease is commoner in men than women.

The arthritis is very painful. It mainly affects joints in the lower part of the body – knees, ankles, feet and toes, although some joints in the upper limbs can be involved too. The foot problems also may include painful inflammation of the deep tissue of the sole, plantar fasciitis, and, later on, formation of a plantar spur of bone beneath the heel bone, the calcaneus (see Chapter 2). The arthritis can also involve the spine, beginning at the lowest level in the sacroiliac joints and spreading slowly upwards exactly as in ankylosing spondylitis. It is these patients who are found to have inherited the characteristic tissue marker for spondylitis, HLA–B27.

With treatment all signs of inflammation subside, but there are usually recurrences in subsequent years, each resembling the original attack of Reiter's disease. In the end there can be some lasting damage to knees and feet and stiffening of the spine. There may also be a thick scaly rash on the soles of the feet, very similar to psoriasis. However, there is no permanent harm to the eyes or the urinary tract.

Treatment. In its acute stage Reiter's disease is treated with rest, drugs for pain relief and an antibiotic such as tetracycline. Within two weeks the signs of acute inflammation have usually settled, but treatment of affected joints needs to continue. This is on the same lines as for rheumatoid arthritis – rest and protection with splint or bandages during the acute stage, after which gentle mobilisation with exercise, physiotherapy or hydrotherapy. A persistently swollen knee will be helped by aspiration of fluid and a steroid injection. Shoes with special cushioned soles will be needed if plantar fasciitis or plantar spur is a problem. Drugs such as gold have no place, nor do steroids other than by local injection.

Treatment for the spine is exactly the same as described for ankylosing spondylitis.

Reactive arthritis

Arthritis in one or more joints may follow infection elsewhere in the body. It is called *reactive arthritis* because it is a complex form of reaction to that infection without the infective organism appearing in the joints themselves. Reiter's disease is one example.

Bowel infections due to various organisms of the food poisoning class (e.g.

Salmonella, E Coli, Campylobacter and others) can be followed by arthritis in one or more joints. This is not as severe as Reiter's disease, recovers without lasting damage and is not subject to recurrences as Reiter's disease is.

Viral infections. The common viral epidemic infections like *rubella* and *mumps* may sometimes cause arthritis is a number of joints (knees, ankles, wrists, fingers). It more often affects adults than children. Although painful at the beginning it subsides within two or three weeks without lasting damage. The changeable nature of epidemic viruses is thought to explain the way in which arthritis may be a feature of an epidemic only occasionally, and then not appear again for some years.

HIV and AIDS may also cause arthritis which can be severe. The impaired immunity present in AIDS carries with it the risk of a dangerous complication of arthritis, whether the arthritis is due to AIDS or to a previous cause – the danger of *septic infection* of a joint. This can be life threatening and requires prompt recognition and treatment with the appropriate antibiotic for the organism infecting the joint.

Rheumatic fever, once so serious among children in the poorer quarters of cities in the 19th and early 20th centuries, has now virtually disappeared in the Western world. However, it is still a problem in some countries e.g. in India and the Far East.

It is commonest in children of school age, and is a reaction to a streptococcal throat infection which occurred some 10 to 14 days previously. Having recovered from the symptoms of the throat infection a child becomes ill again with one or more acutely painful swollen joints and a fever. In a mild case this settles down with rest within a week. In a more serious case the arthritis may move from one joint to another e.g. knee, ankle, elbow, recovering in each in turn, and it may be some weeks before joint pain and fever settle. Small nodules may appear under the skin near the knuckles or elbows; the heart rate is rapid and a heart murmur or friction rub, indicating pericarditis, may be heard. The end result will be recovery with normal joints but a damaged heart, particularly affecting the mitral or aortic valves. A child who has had rheumatic fever once is liable to have further attacks after subsequent streptococcal throat infections, so that prevention is important in order to protect the heart from further damage.

Treatment of the acute attack is with bed rest, splinting or bandaging of painful joints, a course of penicillin to eradicate the streptococcus, and aspirin, which is effective in relieving the joint pain. Bed rest continues if there are signs that the heart is involved, after which convalescence and a return to normal activity follows.

Prevention of further attacks of rheumatic fever means prevention of further streptococcal infections. Fortunately the responsible haemolytic streptococcus remains sensitive to penicillin. Penicillin can be given as twice daily tablets or as once monthly injections and should continue for some years.

Chorea (St Vitus' dance) is related to rheumatic fever in that it too occurs after the same type of streptococcal infection, but after a longer interval. It affects girls rather than boys, causes erratic uncontrollable movements of hands, face and limbs and tearfulness, but does not affect the joints. However, its effect on the heart is the same as rheumatic fever, There is the same liability to subsequent attacks of chorea or of rheumatic fever, affecting the heart. This means that subsequent preventive treatment with penicillin is needed in the same way as after rheumatic fever.

Inflammatory bowel disease

Ulcerative colitis and Crohn's disease (regional ileitis) are important causes of inflammation in the bowel wall which may run a long course or one of intermittent relapses. The main symptom is diarrhoea, sometimes with mucus and blood and, with Crohn's disease, a tendency to form a tender inflammatory mass in the abdomen which threatens obstruction and may need surgery.

Arthritis develops in about 10% of people with either condition, mainly when the disease is at its most active, and improving as the bowel condition improves. The usual form is arthritis of one or more of the larger joints – knee, ankle, elbow – and though painful, it clears up with rest and treatment leaving no permanent damage. There is none of the cartilage erosion seen with rheumatoid arthritis. The arthritis may take another form, affecting the sacroiliac joints, progressing up the spine. In the course of time it produces all the changes of ankylosing spondylitis. About half of these people carry the tissue marker HLA–B27.

Treatment of the limb joints is with rest and, if necessary, splinting in the acute phase, with anti inflammatory drugs such as NSAIDs. After the acute phase is over, gentle mobilisation follows of joint and muscles as described for rheumatoid arthritis. Treatment of the spinal arthritis is as described for ankylosing spondylitis (Chapter 6).

Arthritis in children (Juvenile chronic arthritis)

Fortunately arthritis is not common in children. Even so, as it is estimated to affect about one child in a thousand, this means that there must be some 12000 children with arthritis in the UK. It may start at any age from pre-school years up to 16 and affects more girls than boys. One of its problems is that a very young child may not be able to complain of joint pain; it may only be because a limb is moved in an unusual way that arthritis in, say, knee or shoulder, is spotted.

In its *commonest* form the arthritis involves only a few joints, not more than three or four, beginning in children under school age. A minority also develop inflammation in the eyes – iridocyclitis (uveitis) which is far more serious than the arthritis. With care the arthritis may recover, but the eye trouble continues. It threatens sight by causing adhesions in the iris and damaging the muscles that focus the eye and there is a risk of cataract forming. Regular specialist care is needed. Treatment involves the use of drops to dilate the pupil and cortisone eye drops.

In *boys* arthritis may also involve joints in the feet and in the neck. In later years they may also have low back pain from sacroiliac arthritis, gradually evolving into ankylosing spondylitis.

Older girls may develop arthritis in a number of smaller joints, in hands, feet and wrists, with a symmetrical pattern. This is a childhood form of rheumatoid arthritis and may well be seropositive for the rheumatoid factor. This means that it is likely to continue to be a problem in adult life carrying the risk of leaving stiffened or restricted joint movements. The continuing inflammation in childhood can also have a harmful effect on the growth of neighbouring bones.

Still's disease is a term no longer used in referring to childhood arthritis as a whole. Still's original description was of an unusual and fortunately rare illness beginning with a fever and rash, sometimes with pericarditis making a child ill for some time before the appearance of arthritis. The fever ultimately settles and in most, the joints recover although in some its effect can be damaging.

Treatment

As far as possible the child with arthritis should be treated at home, but it is vital that the management should be supervised regularly by a specialist clinic. Here expert medical and nursing care are available with experienced therapists ready to treat and to give guidance on the details of home care. Specialist advice is on hand for the eyes or for orthopaedic care. If a period in hospital proves necessary schooling can be provided.

As described for rheumatoid arthritis, the essentials of treatment are for resting inflamed joints, with specially made splints as required, relief of pain, followed by careful mobilisation and muscle strengthening exercises taught by the physiotherapist. A flexion deformity that restricts the full movement of a joint must be overcome by patient exercise, massage and use of serial splinting. Hydrotherapy in a warm pool is most helpful.

Drugs: Aspirin is no longer given, but non–steroid anti inflammatory (NSAID) drugs such as ibuprofen or naproxen are safe. If joint inflammation does not subside, certain slow acting drugs are given, as for adults: sulphasalazine, gold injections in small doses, and if necessary, methotrexate, under careful monitoring for possible side effects.

Should a child be left, in the end, with damaged joints and any degree of disability, the greatest care must be taken to give emotional support, maintain morale and encourage what activities are possible. Much help and advice is available from organisations and publications given in the appendix.

6 | Ankylosing Spondylitis

In ankylosing spondylitis low grade inflammation begins at the base of the spine in the sacroiliac joints (Figure 6.1) and spreads very gradually upwards causing aching and stiffness. Ultimately, over a matter of years, the spine may become rigid, the so-called "poker back". It begins most often in young men aged 15 to 30 and less often in young women. Men are three times as often affected as women, in whom the disease is altogether milder.

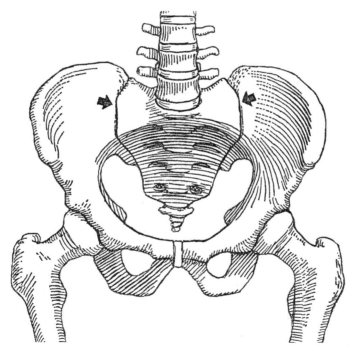

Figure 6.1: The bony pelvis – The sacroiliac joints are indicated; ankylosing spondylitis usually begins here

The inflammation of ankylosing spondylitis begins in a different way from that of rheumatoid arthritis and the other forms of arthritis that we have considered so far. Instead of starting in the lining (synovium) of a joint it starts at places where ligaments, tendons and muscles are attached to bone (entheses). Here lymphocytes and other cells gather and set up a form of inflammation which is long lasting but not very acute. It finally heals by the laying down fibrous tissue; later on this calcifies and finally turns to bone. This process goes on around the margins of the sacroiliac joints (which normally allow very little movement anyway) ending up by fixing those joints. The same happens in the ligaments which surround the margins of the intervertebral discs, the annular ligaments, as well as the small facetal joints between vertebrae and the joints between vertebrae and the twelve pairs of ribs. This has the effect of making the whole spine rigid, right up to the neck (Figure 6.2). The X ray appearance of vertebrae, fused together by fine bridges of bone has been called "bamboo spine"

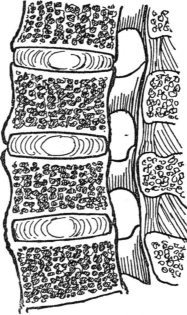

Figure 6.2: Lumbar spine – showing how calcification in ligaments, spreading upwards, fuse the vertebrae together

A similar process in the feet affects the deep fibrous fascia and its attachment to the under side of the heel bone, and the attachment of the Achilles tendon to the top of the heel bone.

In the later stages of the more serious forms of ankylosing spondylitis inflammation develops in some of the bigger limb joints hips, shoulders, knees – and here the process is similar to that of rheumatoid arthritis, eroding cartilage and causing painful restriction of joint movement.

Symptoms and progression are very variable. The start of spondylitis may be so gradual that its presence is not at first recognised. Its presence is explained as "a little back stiffness", yet, after a period of years the end result can be much restriction of back movement or even complete rigidity. In more acute cases there is troublesome low back pain which radiates down the backs of the thighs. This is worst at night, disturbing sleep and causing much stiffness in the morning, with a sense of fatigue. There may be periods of trouble and periods of quiescence, but the inflammation rarely dies out completely.

The result is greatly reduced spinal movement, especially in the lumbar and thoracic areas. All bending and twisting movements are virtually abolished so that it is necessary to move the trunk as a whole from the hips. Neck movements are reduced or finally lost, so that the affected person, instead of turning his head to one side or the other, has to turn his whole body sideways. This creates practical problems with activities such as car driving. Should hip movements become restricted too the situation is really serious, although this is fortunately unusual.

If proper care is not taken in the early stages of ankylosing spondylitis there is a real danger that the spine may become fixed in a bad position, bent forwards. In Figure 6.3 the lumbar and lower thoracic part of the spine is straight, but the upper thoracic, at shoulder level is bent forwards (kyphosis); in compensation for this the neck is bent backwards (extended). Had the neck become fixed when bent forwards the unfortunate patient would have been unable to lift his gaze above the horizontal. Had the lower spine been bent forwards too, matters would have been even worse.

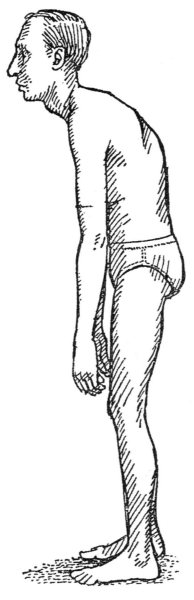

Figure 6.3: Ankylosing spondylitis – There is a danger of a fixed forward flexion deformity, as shown here

Chest expansion is reduced because of the involvement of the joints between the ribs and the spine. This limits the rise and fall of the chest on breathing so that, on taking a deep breath chest expansion is as little as an inch instead of the usual four or five inches. The mechanism of breathing continues satisfactorily through the rise and fall of the diaphragm.

The feet suffer if inflammation involves the fascia lying deeply within the sole – plantar fasciitis – and a bony spur may form at the point of attachment of the fascia beneath the heel bone (see also Chapter 2) This causes discomfort on walking unless a soft padded insole is worn, preferably with strongly soled shoes. Another tender point may be at the rear of the heel bone where the Achilles tendon is attached.

The eyes. A quarter or more of people with ankylosing spondylitis suffer from attacks of inflammation in the iris and in the ciliary body which controls focussing (uveitis). The eyes are painful and vision is blurred. Treatment is with drops to dilate the pupil (mydriatics) in order to avoid adhesions involving the iris, and with cortisone drops to suppress inflammation.

The heart. A small proportion of spondylitic patients, those with the most serious and long standing disease, develop complications involving the heart. The aortic valve becomes inefficient due to weakness and stretching of the wall of the aorta; after each heart beat blood leaks back into the left ventricle, adding to the work of the heart and is a possible cause of heart failure. Surgical valve replacement may be necessary. Another possible complication is failure of conduction of the stimulus which passes within the heart from atrium to ventricle to initiate each beat (heart block). This makes the heart rate drop to a dangerously low level, requiring treatment with a pacemaker.

Inheritance. Ankylosing spondylitis tends to run in families. The explanation is that 95% of all spondylitics carry the tissue marker HLA-B27, inherited from one or other parent. This is a complex molecule, present on the surface of all the body's cells. Its proper name is a "histocompatibility antigen", meaning that it is one of the many tissue markers that must be present in both donor and recipient in transplant surgery if the donor tissue is to be compatible with the recipient.

Because of the consistent association of HLA-B27 with ankylosing spondylitis it has been found, in various populations, that the frequency with which HLA-B27 is present influences the frequency with which spondylitis occurs in that population. For example, in Afro-Caribbean blacks and Australian aborigines HLA-B27 is rarely present, and among them spondylitis is virtually unknown. Some American Indian tribes go to the other extreme, with a high frequency of this tissue marker and of spondylitis.

But this is not the whole story. In European whites (Caucasians) about 8% carry HLA-B27 yet the frequency of spondylitis is under 1%. There must be a trigger factor to which those with the tissue marker are susceptible, causing the start of spondylitis. So far the trigger factor has not been identified, but suspicion points to one or more of the organisms that cause bowel infections. Once the spondylitic process has begun it is capable of becoming self perpetuating, although this does not always happen.

The presence of the tissue marker HLA-B27 is the link between spondylitis and Reiter's disease, psoriasis and inflammatory bowel disease, as explained in Chapter 6. In these conditions the marker is present with a frequency of 30 to 70%.

Treatment

As soon as the diagnosis of ankylosing spondylitis is made it is vital that the patient should be taught the importance of regular exercises in maintaining a good upright posture and preventing the back becoming bent forwards (kyphosis). If the day's activities involve spending time bent over a table or desk then there must be break periods when corrective exercises can be undertaken.

Exercises should concentrate on straightening the back, bending sideways, arching backwards. turning sideways to left and right. Head and neck movements similarly should be in all directions coupled with shoulder and arm movement and deep breathing in time with upwards arm movements, Such a programme of exercises should be carried out at least twice daily for periods of 15 minutes.

Similar movements in a swimming pool or therapy pool are excellent. Some hospitals and clinics arrange that groups of spondylitics attend for back and aerobic exercises and team games in the gymnasium. The existence of active and supportive groups like these is valuable, and so is the National Association for spondylitics (see Appendix).

Pain relief. During periods when the spondylitis is causing pain such vigorous exercises are obviously unsuitable, Rest periods are needed, if necessary fitted in during the working day. In this case care must be taken to see that the back is rested in as straight as posture as possible, on a firm mattress or mat, followed by as much exercise as can be tolerated without pain.

Drugs will be needed for pain relief. Indomethacin (Indocid), ibuprofen (Brufen, Nurofen) and naproxen (Naprosyn) are effective. Overnight pain relief may be given by a bigger dose on retiring, or by a rectal suppository of indomethacin, the effect of which lasts for some hours. In the past, radiotherapy to the spine was much used, and did relieve pain, but this was dangerous in its effect on the bone marrow and is not now used. Similarly the drug phenylbutazone (Butazolidine), though effective was dropped because of harmful side effects.

Surgery as a rule has no place in treatment unless spondylitis has damaged the hip joints or caused severe spinal deformity.

Hip replacement can successfully free the movement of one or both hips if these have become restricted; the liberation in physical activity given to the spondylitic patient by the return of hip movement is immense. Fortunately the "life expectancy" of a modern hip replacement is likely to be as long as that of the patient.

Spinal surgery is rarely needed and is only justified if inadequate treatment or neglect has led to crippling flexion deformity of the spine i.e. bent forward and fixed to such a degree that normal living is badly hampered. It is possible by cutting into the fused vertebral column to realign the back at a somewhat better angle but the operation is hazardous because of the risk of damage to the spinal cord.

7 | Connective tissue diseases

The three conditions described here are all forms of auto immune disease, though in none of them do we fully understand just what starts off this process. In each of them there are inflammatory changes in the walls of blood vessels (vasculitis, arteritis) whose effects are felt in connective tissue in various parts of the body and in some organs. It is this that has led to their being named connective tissue diseases.

Polymyalgia rheumatica

This is an unpleasant illness which affects older adults, causing pain and much stiffness in the shoulders and upper arms and to a less extent the hips and thighs. The patient is almost always over 60 years of age and is more likely to be a woman than a man, the sex ratio being about 3 to 1. It develops over a matter of a few days for no apparent reason. As well as the pain and stiffness in the shoulders and hips the sufferer feels unwell, with loss of energy, loss of appetite and begins to lose weight. A prominent feature is the severe morning stiffness which wears off to some extent during the day. Occasionally there is joint swelling in shoulder, elbow or knee but this ultimately settles down with no after effect. If untreated the illness runs a course of several weeks before slowly subsiding with a gradual return to normal health.

Arteritis. In some patients with polymyalgia a tender thickening develops in certain arteries in the scalp, notably the arteries in the temple, above and in front of the ears. This is due to inflammation in the walls of those arteries and the condition is referred to as cranial or temporal arteritis. If a small section of an affected artery is removed for biopsy, an action which also relieves local pain, a characteristic pattern of inflammation is seen under the microscope in the vessel wall. Unusually large cells are present, giving rise to another name, "giant cell arteritis". For simplicity we shall just use the name "cranial arteritis".

It is now realised that polymyalgia and cranial arteritis are really the same condition in different forms, the latter being the more severe. In cranial arteritis all the unpleasant symptoms of polymyalgia are present, and in polymyalgia there may be arteritis in places that are not apparent. In particular this means that the retinal arteries could be affected threatening blindness in one or both eyes.

For this reason it is important to treat polymyalgia and cranial arteritis promptly and effectively in order to protect the eyes. This is why steroid treatment is almost invariably given.

Treatment. The response to steroid treatment is dramatic. Within a day or two the pain and stiffness of polymyalgia is relieved and the patient begins to feel well again. The tender cranial or temporal arteries lose their tenderness and the visible and palpable swelling in their walls begins to subside. A bigger dose is required for cranial arteritis, e.g. 20 mg daily or more at first, and half this for polymyalgia.

Because steroid treatment carries with it a risk of side effects, particularly in the elderly, it is important that the daily dose should be reduced when possible, but gradually. Steroid treatment should never be stopped suddenly. While steroids are being given the body's own production of steroid by the adrenal glands (in the form of cortisol) is suppressed. If treatment were suddenly withheld, the body would suffer a dangerous state of steroid deficiency until the adrenal glands begin to secrete again. This would cause a drop in blood pressure and a deficiency in sodium and fluid, a form of circulatory collapse.

To avoid this danger, steroid dosage is continued at the initial level until symptoms have fully responded, which may be for some weeks. The daily dosage is then reduced by a small amount and left at that level for another period of weeks and so on. Should symptoms return the dosage may need to be increased again and after a while the gradual reduction begins once more. In many cases the complete withdrawal of steroids may not be possible for one or two years or even more. Once the dose is down to 5 mg prednisone daily the risk of side effects is slight. If it is difficult to reduce to this level other anti inflammatory drugs such as the NSAIDs may be introduced as "steroid sparers".

Systemic lupus

Systemic lupus erythematosus (SLE), to give it its full name, is uncommon in white Europeans but relatively common in black races and orientals. Women are affected much more often than men. It is the most striking and the most intensively studied of the auto immune diseases because of the many auto antibodies that are produced by the patient's own immune system. The predominant antibody acts against DNA itself, and its effects can involve every system in the body.

One characteristic way in which systemic lupus can begin is in a young woman after exposure to sunlight. A rash appears on the face, mainly on the two cheeks, suggesting a "butterfly" distribution and may last for some weeks. Other symptoms appear: pains in joints: some joints may swell, suggesting rheumatoid arthritis. Changes in the blood include anaemia, a reduction in white cells and in blood platelets, which may give rise to bruising and bleeding. Sometimes the causative event is an infection, or the use of certain drugs to which the patient is sensitive, such as sulphonamides. In some patients there may be effects in the lungs, with pleurisy, or the heart, with pericarditis, or the nervous system or the kidneys.

Alarming as this account is, it must be remembered that the majority of cases of systemic lupus are mild and readily treatable, having only one or two of the symptoms mentioned. The important thing is that the nature of the illness should be recognised so that treatment can start.

Treatment needs to be monitored at a specialist clinic so that the extent of the disease can be assessed and treatment regulated accordingly. As a rule the disease can be arrested, or reduced to a minimum, but any sign of a recurrence or flare up should be quickly reported. Unexplained fatigue is a warning sign.

In many cases the anti malarial drugs chloroquin (Nivaquin) or hydroxychloroquin (Plaquenil) are effective. If they are given over a matter of months, periodic eye checks are recommended as very occasionally they may harm the retina or the cornea. Should anti malarial drugs not control the disease, steroids are given in the same way as described under polymyalgia. For some of the more serious forms of systemic lupus an unduly high dosage level of steroids can be avoided by the use of immuno suppressive drugs such as azathioprin or methotrexate, both of which need careful supervision.

The patient with systemic lupus must be warned about circumstances or drugs that might cause a flare up. These include skin exposure to sunlight, so that suitable protective clothing should be worn and sunscreen lotions used, and sulphonamide drugs and some antibiotics.

Patients may be reassured by contacting the national support group which offers practical advice to people with systemic lupus. (See Appendix).

Scleroderma (Systemic Sclerosis)

Scleroderma is a rare condition, affecting the skin and flesh of the fingers and face, mainly in women. Very gradually the finger tips become slightly shrunken and firmer. To some extent the whole of the fingers are affected so that finger movements are a little restricted, without involvement of the joints. Similar changes slowly evolve in the lower part of the face and around the lips which become less full and less supple with a little wrinkling of the flesh around the mouth.

Almost always the changes of scleroderma are preceded, probably for years, by attacks of vascular spasm in the fingers – Raynaud's phenomenon. Scleroderma is part of a wider disorder, systemic sclerosis, which may involve other parts of the body, particularly the oesophagus, lungs, heart and kidneys.

The basic cause of these changes is a slowly progressive thickening in the walls of small blood vessels which reduces the blood flow. Some vessels become blocked altogether. The result is shrinking and fibrosis in the tissues that are deprived of their proper blood supply.

Raynaud's phenomenon is very common in girls and young women. On brief exposure of the hands to cold there is spasm in the small arteries in one or more fingers, which go white and "dead", later turning blue and finally pink as the blood flow returns on warming. Smoking may also bring on this spasm, and sometimes it is a response to emotion. Severe repeated attacks may lead to sores around the finger tips which are slow to heal. Many women find that these attacks lessen or stop as they grow older. Only in a small minority is Raynaud's phenomenon the precursor to rheumatoid arthritis, systemic lupus or scleroderma.

Systemic sclerosis is the manifestation elsewhere in the body of the same process that produces scleroderma in the fingers and face. It may first become apparent in the oesophagus, causing some difficulty in swallowing or reflux of stomach acid as happens with hiatus hernia. This is relieved by antacids or by drugs that reduce the secretion of stomach acid. Other troubles that may follow, and then only after some years, are changes in the lung blood vessels, or in the kidney, which may cause raised blood pressure, and in the heart.

Treatment of *Raynaud's phenomenon* is, in the first place, preventative. This means protecting the hands and face from undue exposure to cold; proper clothing should be worn to conserve body heat as a whole, and gloves should be worn in cold weather. Immersion of the hands in cold water should be avoided. There should be no smoking. Certain drugs may be taken to assist the circulation such as nifedipine (Adalat) or nicotinic acid. The herbal remedy Prickly Ash Bark, taken internally is of help.

The treatment of *scleroderma* includes the measures recommended for Raynaud's phenomenon. In addition it is helpful regularly to massage the fingers and face with an emollient cream, with the aim of delaying the thickening and hardening process of fibrosis in the skin.

Treatment for *Systemic Sclerosis* is determined by the organ or system which is affected. If it is the oesophagus, producing swallowing difficulties or acid reflux, treatment is with antacids, or drugs to reduce the stomach's secretion of acid, as has already been mentioned. Involvement of the heart may require drug treatment to regularise the rhythm, which may be disturbed, and digitalis if the heart muscle function is impaired. If blood pressure is raised as a result of kidney involvement there are many remedies available of which the most appropriate is probably an ACE inhibitor.

There is a national association for people suffering from Raynaud's phenomenon or from scleroderma, to whom members may apply for further practical advice (see Appendix).

8 | Crystal arthritis: Gout and Pseudogout

The dramatic nature of an attack of gout in the foot has meant that it was recognised and described centuries ago. Hippocrates himself made observations on gout which still hold true today. More recently, in the 18th and 19th centuries politically motivated cartoons caricatured gout sufferers as self indulgent aristocrats addicted to rich food and wine – a social distinction that is now no longer true (Figure 8.1).

We know that gout is associated with an increase in uric acid in the blood and that an acute attack is brought on by the release of urate crystals in a joint. We have also learned that crystals other than urate can sometimes provoke identical attacks, a condition that has been named pseudo gout – although the victim is likely to describe his attack as anything but pseudo.

Gout is commoner in men than in women and tends to run in families. There are considerable racial variations in the incidence of gout; it is virtually unknown in black people, but is frequent in Polynesians and so, in New Zealand, is commonly seen in Maoris. This is an indication that inherited tendencies, racial or familial, are more significant than diet in determining who will suffer from gout.

Blood uric acid. The level of uric acid in the blood has an important bearing on the manifestations of gout. The level is a little higher, on average, in men than in women, 6 or 7mg per 100ml compared with 5mg. Uric acid is a waste product, the end result of the chemical breakdown of certain constituents of protein, nucleic acids. The level in the blood is determined by the balance between the rate of production of uric acid and the rate of its excretion by the kidneys. Excess production and slow excretion of uric acid therefore both have a part to play in raising the blood level. Another factor influencing the onset of an attack is the local chemical relationship between the blood and the joint tissues and

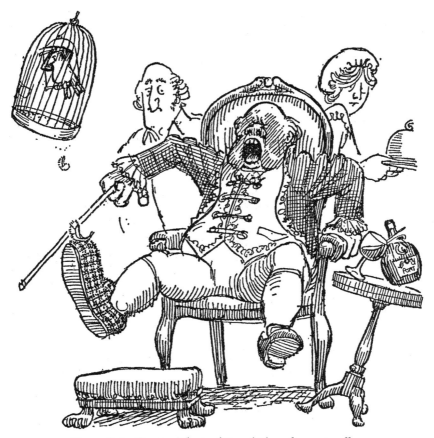

Figure 8.1: Gout — The traditional idea of a gout sufferer

fluid. This can determine whether uric acid can remain painlessly in solution, or crystallise as sodium urate in the joint fluid, thereby setting up a painful reaction. It may also explain why gout tends to attack a joint that is already slightly damaged.

Excess production of uric acid can have a number of possible causes. Serious injury or infection, major surgery or any wasting disease induce a breakdown of body tissues; the protein component of this breakdown is the source of the extra uric acid. Some blood diseases, such as leukaemia and its treatment liberate quantities of uric acid from the turnover and destruction of nucleated cells. Psoriasis, if extensive, liberates uric acid from the quantities of skin cells that are produced and destroyed.

Excesses of food and drink, too, may bring on an attack in a person already liable to suffer from gout. The foods most likely to do this are high protein foods containing many nucleated cells: red meat, liver, kidneys, sweetbread and fish roe. Some kinds of drink have a reputation for provoking gout, such as port, Madeira and Burgundy.

Crystals appearing in joint fluid, whether of urate or of a different type, provoke an immediate inflammatory reaction. This floods the joint with white cells, polymorphs, which engulf the crystals. But in so doing, the polymorphs themselves are liable to be destroyed, releasing the powerful enzymes that they carry, and this is considered to be largely the cause of the pain. The associated increase in blood flow to the joint explains the heat, redness and swelling of the inflammation.

An acute attack of gout typically begins in the night, and the joint most often affected is the joint at the base of the big toe. This may be because this is the joint which in most people is likely already to have been damaged by osteoarthritis. Very quickly pain and swelling build up to a peak. The weight of the bedclothes becomes intolerable and the sufferer finds that he must rest the leg up, slightly elevated and uncovered. It was for this reason the "gout stools" of the 18th century were designed. Without specific treatment the pain and swelling might continue for a week before subsiding, although correct treatment today will relieve pain within a matter of hours. Sometimes other joints are affected – the ankle, knee, wrist or elbow.

Subsequent course. Once the acute attack is over the joint returns practically to normal and there may be no further signs of gout for months or years. But if more attacks follow this is damaging to the affected joint or joints. Deposits of urate form in the articular cartilage or the underlying bone, producing erosions of bone which on X-ray look like those seen in rheumatoid arthritis, only bigger, damaging the joint permanently. Further deposits of urate may be laid down elsewhere in the body; these are called tophi.

Tophi are only formed after gout has been active or inadequately treated for a number of years. They are chalky white deposits occurring in or near joints, under the skin near the point of the elbow, in the cartilage of the ear and elsewhere. Sometimes the white deposit ulcerates through the skin.

The kidneys are often affected in men with long standing gout. The reason is the amount of urate that the kidneys have to excrete. The act of concentrating the fluid that passes through the kidney in the formation of urine, can cause urate to deposit within the kidney either as crystals or as tophus–like deposits. Sometimes a urate stone is formed and may be passed down into the bladder with much pain. In the course of time kidney function becomes impaired and can be a cause of high blood pressure or even of kidney failure. Kidney damage can also contribute to delay in the excretion of uric acid. Another reason for delay in excretion sometimes is a reaction to treatment with thiazide diuretics; prolonged use of this type of diuretic can, in a few patients, lead to development of gout.

The programme of treatment of gout must be planned with care if the kidneys are known to be affected, because treatment, by releasing urate from deposits in the body may run the risk of contributing to further deposits in the kidney. It is possible to avoid this.

Treatment

Acute gout. A traditional and effective remedy is *colchicine*, which is derived from the autumn crocus. It is taken in the form of a tablet of 0.5 mg every two hours for 8 doses or more, but by this time it may produce side effects, diarrhoea or sickness. For this reason, in older people it is better given at longer intervals, of four hours.

Indomethacine (Indocid) and *naproxen* (Naprosyn) and other anti inflammatory drugs are also quickly effective; they need to be continued for some days. Phenylbutazone (Butazolidine) was much used in recent years but, though very effective it was withdrawn because of harmful side effects. Surprisingly, aspirin is best avoided in acute gout as it may raise the blood level of uric acid.

If the attack of gout was an isolated event, brought on by circumstances that are unlikely to recur, further drug treatment may be considered unnecessary. However, two precautions should be taken. It is advisable for the patient to have available an emergency supply of colchicine or indomethacine, and also to consider his diet.

Diet. Attention to diet is important if there has been more than one attack of gout or if there is a known family tendency. The foods to be avoided, as mentioned above, are those with a high protein content, especially if rich in nucleic acids This means red meat, liver, kidney, sweetbread, sardines, and fortified wines such as port, Madeira and sherry. Any overindulgence in alcohol is unwise. In hot climates it is important to maintain a good fluid intake, so as to assist kidney function.

A change to a vegetarian diet is not necessary, but would certainly help a gouty subject by "playing safe", It is worth remembering too that celery and celery seed have a traditional reputation as a remedy for gout.

Uricosuric drugs. These are drugs which act on the kidneys making them increase their output of uric acid, thereby helping to prevent a recurrence of gout. They are probenecid (Benemid) and sulphinpyrazone (Anturan). Either of them can be used for long term daily treatment. However, they should not be given during an acute attack, and when they are introduced for the first time they may indeed provoke an acute attack. For this reason colchicine or indomethacin are given in addition to the uricosuric drug for the first week or two. They are also unsuitable for treating a gouty person who already has damaged kidneys as their action could make the kidney condition worse.

Allopurinol (Zyloric) is the best drug for long term treatment of the gouty person who is liable to acute attacks, has tophi or deposits in bone or who has kidney damage. The action of allopurinol is to block the final stage in the chemical chain reaction which leads up to the formation of uric acid. The process is stopped at xanthine, the precursor of uric acid, which the kidneys can excrete safely. By taking allopurinol daily over a long period the gouty deposits are gradually mobilised and excreted without harming the kidneys, and the patient is protected from acute attacks. One precaution is necessary: when allopurinol is first given, it too may provoke an acute attack of gout, and so for the first week or two, colchicine or indomethacin is given in addition.

Pseudo gout

Gout-like attacks can be due to crystals of a different kind, *Calcium pyrophosphate* (CPPD). Such attacks are sometimes referred to as CPPD gout, as distinct from urate gout.

Chondrocalcinosis is the condition in which this may occur. The crystals in this case are released into the joint, not from the blood, but from deposits of CPPD in cartilage. Because of its calcium content CPPD shows up on X ray; it is seen as a fine shadowy line within the articular cartilage of the knee or shoulder joint, in the semilunar cartilage (meniscus) of the knee and in relation to other joints. Its presence there is painless, at least initially, and it may be a chance finding when an X ray is taken of an older person. However, it is thought likely to predispose to osteoarthritis, especially in the knees. Occasionally it gives rise to an attack of acute joint pain and swelling in the knee, lasting for some days, just as in urate gout. The true diagnosis can only be made with certainty by drawing off a sample of joint fluid during the attack and examining it under the microscope. The crystals of urate are fine and needle like, while those of CPPD are shorter and blunter. When examined with polarised light there are other differences between the two types of crystal.

We do not yet understand the cause of chondrocalcinosis. It may be due to an inherited tendency, for in some rare cases there is a strong family history with symptoms beginning in early adult life, making a parallel with urate gout. But as a rule the condition arises sporadically, mainly in older adults, sometimes giving trouble and sometimes not.

Treatment of an acute attack of CPPD gout is similar to that of urate gout. Colchicine is rather less effective so that reliance has to be on anti inflammatory drugs like indomethacin, naproxen or ibuprofen. For very severe pain a steroid injection into the joint brings quick relief. When there is florid osteoarthritis as well as CPPD gout in the knee, surgical replacement may be considered.

Other crystals

Hydroxyapatite which is a normal constituent of bone, may sometimes form deposits in the region of joints, particularly the shoulder and near tendon sheaths. The appearance of these crystals in the shoulder joint itself, or in a nearby bursa gives rise to sudden severe pain. It is best treated with a local steroid injection.

9 | Bone disorders

Our bones are the strongest and most enduring parts of our body. Yet, like all living tissues, they are subject to a continual but gradual process of absorption and renewal. In the adult, 10% of the body's bone is renewed each year, and in the child, a much greater proportion. This enables bone to be remodelled and reinforced so as to meet the stresses of everyday activity.

The greater part, 80%, of skeletal mass is in the strong outer shell or cortex of our bones, and the remainder is in the inner, finer, strands of cancellous bone (Figure 9.1) which is where the bone marrow is.

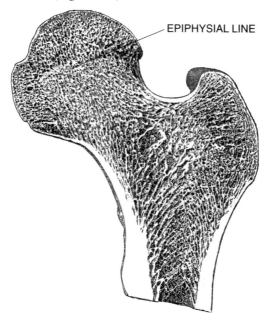

Figure 9.1: Head of femur – Cross section of a normal femoral head, showing the outer cortex and the inner cancellous bone

Structure. The basic ground substance of bone is collagen, the same protein that forms connective tissue throughout the body. This is impregnated with calcium combined with the crystalline substance hydroxyapatite. Normal bone formation requires that calcium and phosphorus should be made available from the diet and that vitamin D should be present to enable the chemical process to go ahead. The composition of bone is also influenced by hormones from the thyroid and parathyroid glands, by the sex hormones, oestrogen and testosterone, and by corticosteroids i.e. cortisone and its relatives. Lodged within bone are the important cells which control the removal and the new formation of bone; both are continually active.

Development. When we are born our skeleton is made largely of cartilage, but in many bones small centres of ossification are already present. Throughout childhood further centres appear and by the time that adult stature is reached the replacement of cartilage by bone is complete. In childhood limb bones are able to grow in length because they have one main centre of bone formation in the shaft, with a small centre of bone formation like a cap at each end (the epiphysis). When growth is completed each cap fuses with the shaft so that no further growth in length is possible.

Just as muscles grow strong through exercise, so bones grow strong in response to the stresses imposed by physical activity – supporting the body's weight, sustaining the extra forces applied by bodily movement, and providing a firm base for muscular attachments. Physical and sporting activity in childhood and youth, combined with good nutrition, are therefore beneficial in the building up of healthy bones. The body's maximum bone mass is achieved by the age of 30, remaining constant for some 20 years and diminishing after that. The experience of prolonged weightlessness in astronauts has taught us that removing the stimulus of the natural stresses imposed by gravity results in the skeleton becoming weaker and losing calcium, giving rise to osteoporosis.

Osteoporosis

Osteoporosis is a condition in which the mass of bone in relation to its volume is significantly reduced, so making the bones less dense and weaker. This reduction in strength carries with it the risk of fracture, even after minor injury.

After reaching its peak in mid life, the mass and strength of bone diminishes at different rates in the two sexes. In women this diminution is greatest during the 5 to 10 years that follow the menopause and is related to the reduction in secretion of oestrogen by the ovaries. If the ovaries have already been removed by surgery or destroyed by disease, producing a premature menopause, the effect on bone is greater because the decline has started at an earlier age. In men the decline in bone strength is much more gradual, in parallel with the gradual falling off in secretion of testosterone with age.

The result is that osteoporosis and the consequent risk of fracture in older people is greater in women than in men. Spontaneous fractures of vertebrae are ten times as common in older women as in men, and fractures of the neck of the femur three times as common. There is considerable individual variation. Those who have built up strong bones in early adult life, and who maintain a physically active life style are much less likely to suffer from osteoporosis in later years. There are racial variations too: Afro-Caribbean black people tend to have very strong bones and rarely develop osteoporosis.

The most common sites of fractures due to osteoporosis are in the vertebrae, the neck of the femur, and the lower end of the radius just above the wrist (Colles fracture). In the spine, one or more vertebral bodies may gradually give way without pain so that the affected person may lose height by some inches in the course of time. This is usually accompanied by rounding (kyphosis) of the upper back, with the curvature known as "Dowager's hump" (Figure 9.2). Sometimes the collapse of a vertebral body is a sudden very painful event, occurring without warning and without any particular trauma. With rest and analgesics the pain subsides; such fractures heal satisfactorily, although the wedge shaped deformity of the collapsed vertebral body will remain.

Fracture of the neck of femur is often the result of a fall, or an unexpected jolt, as when "missing a step" at the bottom of a stairway. With expert surgical treatment by pinning and good aftercare a satisfactory result is usually achieved, but there are dangers for the elderly

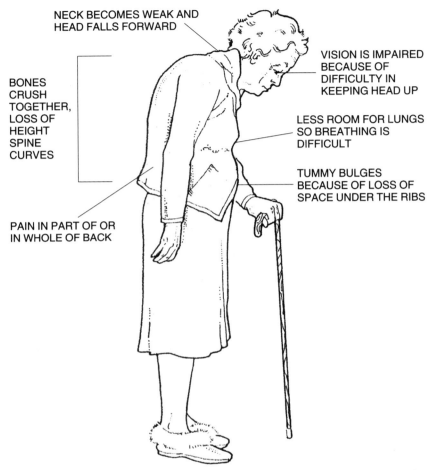

NECK BECOMES WEAK AND
HEAD FALLS FORWARD

BONES
CRUSH
TOGETHER,
LOSS OF
HEIGHT
SPINE
CURVES

VISION IS IMPAIRED
BECAUSE OF
DIFFICULTY IN
KEEPING HEAD UP

LESS ROOM FOR LUNGS
SO BREATHING IS
DIFFICULT

TUMMY BULGES
BECAUSE OF LOSS OF
SPACE UNDER THE RIBS

PAIN IN PART OF OR
IN WHOLE OF BACK

Figure 9.2: Osteoporosis – The "dowager's hump" is due to partial collapse of upper vertebrae

patient, such as chest infections and thrombosis which are potentially life threatening.

X-ray reveals the presence of osteoporosis because it shows that bones appear less dense than normal. However, it is difficult to judge the severity of osteoporosis on X-ray appearance alone. The technique of *bone densitometry*, available in specialist clinics, makes it possible to measure the degree of osteoporosis, to follow its progression year by year, and to assess the response to treatment.

Causes. The main cause of *generalised* osteoporosis is the effect of ageing, accelerated by oestrogen withdrawal after the menopause. Long term treatment with corticosteroids is another important cause, when given for rheumatoid arthritis, asthma or other reasons, and this effect can be added to that of age and the menopause. Additional contributory factors are smoking and alcoholism. Some people have a poor dietary intake of calcium because of a lifelong aversion to milk. It may be that this is due to an unrecognised inborn deficiency of the enzyme lactase, which is responsible for the digestion of lactose, the sugar of milk. Without this enzyme lactose ferments and produces intestinal pain and colic. The missing enzyme can be provided in tablet form, enabling the affected person to take milk and milk products without discomfort, or it can be used to treat milk so as to reduce its content of lactose.

Local osteoporosis can also occur due to disuse, as in a paralysed limb. Lesser degrees of local osteoporosis affect bone next to a chronically inflamed joint, as in the finger bones in people with rheumatoid arthritis; it results from a combination of disuse and the increased blood flow in the region of the inflamed joint.

Management

Prevention is by far the best approach. Ideally, as indicated above, this begins in childhood with good *nutrition* and healthy physical activity. In later life prevention implies continuing regular *exercise* e.g. walking for 30 minutes daily and maintaining a good intake of *calcium* e.g. 1000 to 1500mg daily. A pint of milk contains about 750mg calcium. Other good sources are milk products, green vegetables, shellfish, and sardines. The normal adult requirement of vitamin D, officially set at 400 units daily, is met by a normal diet, but if necessary can easily be obtained, with vitamin A, in capsules of fish liver oil or as a combined supplement with calcium in tablet form. Excessive intake of vitamin D should be avoided as, after a time it can lead to abnormal deposition of calcium in the body and a number of toxic symptoms.

Treatment is necessary for women who have had a premature menopause, for those who have already suffered a fracture due to osteoporosis and for those with a significant degree of osteoporosis shown on bone densitometry.

Hormone replacement therapy (HRT) provides oestrogen with a small amount of progestogen either in the form of a daily tablet or as an implant. It is usually continued for 5 years or longer, but this is a matter for individual decision. It reduces the risks of fracture and of coronary disease and abolishes many of the symptoms of the menopause such as hot flushes. However, the possibility remains that continuing HRT for over ten years may increase the risk of breast cancer. This has not yet been definitely established.

Calcium supplements by themselves are not sufficient to correct osteoporosis although they can slow down its progress. They are certainly helpful when taken in conjunction with HRT or as a preventative against osteoporosis. A daily intake of 1000 to 1500mg is advisable. There are many forms of calcium supplement such as those which combine it with vitamin D, or with magnesium, as Dolomite.

Other treatments, when necessary, are available from clinics specialising in osteoporosis. Biphosphonate (Editronate) slows down the process of bone absorption; anabolic steroids promote bone formation, but tend to have a masculinising effect and fluoride may have a place in hardening bone. These all require medical supervision

In the home. The person with osteoporosis must take extra care to avoid falls and accidents which could cause a fracture. The commonest place for an accident being in the home, this means paying close attention to danger points. These include the edges of carpets and mats, trailing electric flex or telephone leads, stairs, dark corners, pets underfoot etc. Much helpful information on such practical points, and other advice is available from the National Osteoporosis Society (See Appendix).

Vitamin D deficiency

Rickets. This is a condition virtually unknown in this country today, although commonly seen in undernourished children living in poverty in our crowded cities a century or more ago. Today it is only seen in third world conditions of poverty. Its cause is deficiency of vitamin D resulting in inadequate calcification and weakening growing bones.

The most obvious signs of childhood rickets are in the legs, giving rise to "knock knees" or its opposite, bandy legs or even curvature of leg bones. In the chest weakening of the ribs in infants leads to the rib cage being drawn in around the lower chest. There are swellings at the end of the ribs where they join the breast bone, giving the appearance of the so called "rickety rosary". There is muscular weakness too, and bone tenderness.

Vitamin D (calciferol) is a natural component of milk and milk products and there are copious supplies in fish liver oil. It is also formed in the skin by the action of sunlight on cholesterol. Rickets is therefore due to a combination of a diet poor in vitamin D and also lack of exposure of the skin to sunlight.

Treatment. Dietary deficiencies must be corrected by ensuring an adequate daily intake of foods containing vitamin D and calcium, and there may well of course be other deficiencies too. The old fashioned remedy was cod-liver oil, loathed by children, more acceptably replaced today by a capsule of halibut liver oil. The daily requirement of 400 international units is quite sufficient. There is danger of toxicity in taking high doses of the vitamin over long periods.

Osteomalacia

This is the adult equivalent of childhood rickets. The cause is essentially the same – deficiency of vitamin D – but the manifestations are rather different. In the UK it is sometimes seen in poor immigrants from third world countries whose diet and life style make them liable to vitamin D deficiency in the diet and to avoidance of exposure of the skin to sunlight. Osteomalacia has also in the recent past been found in elderly residents in institutions living on an inadequate diet and spending most of their time indoors or in bed. Another possible cause is malabsorption due to long standing bowel disease such as adult coeliac disease, or after surgery on the stomach or bowel.

Weakening of bones in osteomalacia causes partial fractures in various places – in the vertebrae, the pelvis, or in the limb bones. This causes pain which is sometimes wrongly attributed to arthritis, but unlike arthritis it is pain that is not entirely associated with movement, and does not cause stiffness. An X-ray will show the characteristic fractures, which appear as breaks in the surface of a bone without going through its full width (pseudo fractures, or Looser's zones). A bone scan is also helpful. Often these are found in the lower parts of the pelvis, the pubis and ischium, in which case the pain they cause may well be blamed on hip arthritis.

Treatment is simple once osteomalacia has been recognised. It means provision of a correct diet and the addition of vitamin D supplements. It is safest to give rather more than for childhood rickets e.g. 1600 units daily. If faulty absorption of nutrients is due to an intestinal disorder, this will need to be investigated and if possible corrected.

Paget's disease

In Paget's disease a bone or part of a bone undergoes a structural change in which there is excessive absorption followed by faulty rebuilding of bone. The affected area is often expanded in size and may be weakened with a risk of fracture. The blood flow is much increased making the bone feel warm. The cause of Paget's disease is not known, though a viral agent is considered possible.

It is common in older people of either sex: it is rarely seen under 50 years of age, but 10% of those over 80 are found to have these changes in one or more of their bones. They may well be unaware of this, for in most cases it is painless. The bones affected are the skull, the spine and limb bones. In the skull the forehead may become rather more prominent, with a slight increase in the size of the head. As the bone expands it may cause headache and pressure on the acoustic nerve causing deafness. In the spine Paget's disease can cause collapse of a vertebral body and also pressure on a spinal nerve or even on the spinal cord. In the lower leg the changes in the shape of the tibia, which becomes thickened, expanded and slightly curved have given it the name "sabre tibia".

If an area of bone close to a joint is involved, such as the lower end of the femur the function of a joint is affected, contributing to osteoarthritis, in this case, of the knee.

X-ray clearly shows the abnormal bone patterning in affected areas , and biochemical tests confirm that bone is being reabsorbed and rebuilt to an abnormal degree.

Treatment. Fortunately there are effective treatments which can arrest these changes in bone. Biphosphonate (Editronate), taken by mouth with a calcium supplement slows down the process of reabsorption and allows healing and strengthening of bone to occur. Calcitonin too is effective; this is a hormone derived from the thyroid gland.

10 | Complementary medicine and diet

Public interest in the various forms of complementary medicine has greatly increased in recent years and continues to grow. At least a quarter of the UK population make use of one or more of these therapies. The same is true of other countries, and in some, for example France and Germany, the proportion is considerably higher.

The attitude of the medical profession has changed from outright rejection to acceptance, tempered often by tolerant scepticism. In a survey held in London half of the GP's questioned were prepared to refer patients to qualified practitioners of some complementary therapies. One London hospital has set up a complementary medicine clinic in its premises and finds that this attracts more clients than were expected for acupuncture, osteopathy and homoeopathy.

Many sufferers from rheumatism and arthritis are among those attending complementary practitioners with benefit. But in view of the serious nature of many rheumatic complaints it is important that such therapies should truly be complementary to conventional medical care and not a substitute or alternative to it. Ideally complementary and orthodox medical care should together form the basis for holistic care of the individual patient.

Diet

It hardly seems right to consider diet under the heading of complementary medicine, for food and nutrition are an essential part of all our lives. But most patients with rheumatism or arthritis ask for advice on diet; as well as turning to their doctor they often seek further, from a dietician, naturopath or other therapist.

Many dietary recommendations have been offered as a help or as a cure for rheumatic disorders, but clearly the idea of "cure-all diet" is an over simplification. Different rheumatic disorders call for different advice and individual patients vary considerably in their medical state and their nutritional needs.

A dietary programme that helps one patient may be without benefit to another. This has particularly proved to be the case with rheumatoid arthritis; a small minority of patients have been found to be intolerant of or allergic to certain items of food and to be helped by omitting them from their diet. This led to the theory that their intestinal lining was abnormally permeable to relatively complex food substances which could act as allergens and start up the disease. But the majority of patients with rheumatoid arthritis show no sign of such a food allergy.

The story of the Dong diet, which had a great following, is a good example of the difficulties that arise. Dr Dong, when he developed arthritis, firmly believed that a return to the Chinese "poor man's diet" of his youth would cure him – a diet rich in seafood, vegetables and rice, avoiding meat, dairy products, herbs, spices and alcohol.

He made a dramatic recovery, wrote a best selling book about it, and his advice was widely followed. However, when a careful test compared a group of patients on the Dong diet with a control group over a period of 10 weeks, there was no difference between the responses to the two diets.

The best plan is to recommend a basically healthy diet in the light of today's knowledge, and to modify it as necessary according to the nature of the rheumatic disorder and the individual patient's needs and idiosyncracies.

How can we summarise a "basically healthy diet"? It should provide sufficient *protein* to supply the body's needs for tissue repair and growth. For most of us the main source of protein is in the form of meat, milk and dairy products; these give us first class protein which provides amino acids in the proportion best suited to our needs. But this is not essential, for vegetarians and vegans can very well obtain their protein from grains, pulses, nuts and soya, although the amino acid yield is not quite so efficient and vegans are advised to ensure an extra source of vitamin B12.

Carbohydrates supply energy needs largely from their ultimate breakdown into glucose, the body's basic source of chemical energy. On the whole our consumption of glucose and sucrose is excessive as they provide nothing more than "empty calories". It is far better to obtain our carbohydrates in their natural form, as vegetable, fruit and grain; in this form they also give us vitamins, minerals and roughage.

Fats are needed to provide our body's insulation, for cell wall structure, as an energy source and for many derivatives, including the fat soluble vitamins A and D. But we are warned of the dangers of taking too much fat in forms containing saturated fatty acids, contributing to coronary and arterial disease. Fats from fish and vegetable sources with their unsaturated fatty acids are safer for us in this respect.

Ideally, a balanced diet on the principles indicated will give us our necessary nutrients, vitamins and minerals, but for various reasons our daily food is all too often far from ideal. This is too big a subject to be dealt with here, and further reading is advised from the books and sources mentioned in the appendix.

Special dietary needs

Osteoarthritis. Here it is important to avoid becoming overweight, especially if weight bearing joints are affected. This means that foods bringing unnecessary calories must be reduced, mainly carbohydrates and fats, paying attention to quality while reducing quantity. Many people with osteoarthritis are elderly, and they will need a good intake of calcium and possibly vitamin D, in which they are sometimes deficient. A good policy for the older patient would be periodically to take a supplement of calcium with vitamin D.

Gout. Dietary precautions for the gout sufferer were described in Chapter 8. This means moderation in purine-rich foods: red meat, liver, kidney, sweetbread, roe, and with certain drinks: port, Madeira, red wine, beers and stout. Total avoidance of these foods is rarely necessary, as long term treatment with allopurinol is effective. One warning for the gout patient is this: to miss a main meal such as lunch, and later to indulge in alcoholic drinks on an empty stomach is a recipe for provoking an attack of gout. Another warning is to avoid dehydration in hot weather or in a hot climate, which, again, may provoke an attack.

Rheumatoid arthritis. As already mentioned, a small proportion of people with rheumatoid arthritis are *intolerant* of an item of diet, improving when it is avoided, worsening when it is taken again. Food items that have been incriminated in this way include: corn, wheat, rye, oats, bacon and oranges. In some cases the offending component may be gluten. The simplest approach is for the patient to note carefully if there is any regular association between symptoms and any particular item of diet, and then to seek confirmation by a period of exclusion of that item, checking whether reintroduction brings back the symptoms. Without good evidence of intolerance, dietary restrictions can be an unnecessary complication to daily life. The same possibility of food intolerance should be considered in the case of systemic lupus.

Fasting for a few days has been shown to relieve inflammation when rheumatoid arthritis or any similar form of arthritis is in an active phase. This is not the result of avoiding food intolerance, but appears to be because reducing all nutrients reduces the raw materials from which inflammatory agents are made. Such a fast should not be for more than a week and should be made under medical supervision. Extra rest is needed during a fast, and fluid intake must be maintained. Fruit and vegetable juices are valuable.

Fish oil supplements help to reduce the inflammatory process in active rheumatoid arthritis. This is due to their content of unsaturated fatty acids of the n-3 class (EPA and DHA). By their presence in the body these compete with other unsaturated fatty acids which are the source of inflammatory chemical agents. However, a fairly large daily dose is necessary (EPA 15 grams) which is expensive.

Evening primrose oil has a similar though milder anti–inflammatory effect as the fish oils through its content of gamma–linolenic acid (GLA). Up to 10 capsules of 0.5 gram daily are necessary and, again, this is expensive.

Green lipped mussel. This too has a mild anti–inflammatory effect and is safe, although some studies have failed to confirm the claims made for it.

Vitamin supplements. In the presence of a chronic inflammatory or debilitating disease the body's needs for protective antioxidant agents is increased. These are vitamin C, which is water soluble, and vitamin E, which is fat soluble, and selenium. No precise recommendations can be made about dosage, but a reasonable daily amount would be 0.5 to 1 gram of vitamin C, 20mg of vitamin E and 100 micrograms of selenium. They can be obtained in a combined tablet form, or less expensively, in individual powder form (see Appendix) Some people may prefer to obtain vitamin supplements in a more natural form as derived from rose hips, blackcurrant or other fruit sources.

Herbal medicine

This is the oldest form of medicine, for herbs have always been with us. Up to a century ago the physician, pharmacist and herbalist shared a common knowledge of herbs and their virtues. Today the growth of scientific medicine and the development of powerful and effective drugs had led to a widespread wish that we should not forget the natural origin of many of our medicines – the herbs themselves.

A wide range of therapeutic herbs is available to us from herbalists and health food shops. They come either as single herb preparations or in combination, and in all cases have to meet standards of quality that are regulated by law. This requires that they should be safe for over-the-counter (OTC) sale, intended for self medication.

A number of herbs have a long standing reputation for relieving rheumatic symptoms. Some are simply pain relievers, some are anti inflammatory and others relieve muscle spasm or nerve pain. Many have been tested by the critical clinical methods of today and their efficacy has been confirmed. In some cases a test may have proved negative in spite of a herb's long standing reputation; perhaps our tests are sometimes too strict, or expect too rapid a response, for the healing effect of many herbal remedies is gentle and slow.

Brief descriptions of some of the herbs known for their use in rheumatism and arthritis are as follows:

Black Cohosh Cimicifuga racemosa
This plant comes from North America where it is known to the Indians as black snakeroot. A powdered extract is made from the dried root or rhizome. This contains chemicals that are related to aspirin and others that have an oestrogen–like action. It is used for relief of joint pain and inflammation and for back pain due to osteoarthritis and ankylosing spondylitis. Its oestrogen–like action means that it has a role in treating

painful menstruation, and menopausal symptoms, but it should not be given during pregnancy.

Bogbean *Menyanthes trifoliata*
This is the marsh trefoil. An extract of its dried leaves is used as a bitter, stimulating appetite, and it also has an aperient effect. It eases rheumatic pain and stiffness and is sometimes combined with Black Cohosh and Celery seed.

Celery seeds *Apium graveolens*
Celery itself or an infusion made from its crushed seeds relieves muscular stiffness and pain. As it also has a mild diuretic action it has been used in the treatment of gout.

Devil's Claw *Harpagophytum procumbens*
This plant grows in the sandy desert like soil of SW Africa and is known as "grapple plant" because of its woody fruit covered with claw like barbs. The root produces tubers which yield the active principles, given as a dried powder for relief of pain and stiffness in soft tissue rheumatism, and for arthritis.

Feverfew *Tanacetum parthenii*
This plant grows readily in our gardens. Preparations from its leaves have been used for relief of fever and for headaches and today it is given as a prophylactic against migraine. It is also taken for back and joint pain. Its rather bitter leaves traditionally can be consumed in a sandwich.

Guiacum *Lignum vitae*
This is an evergreen tree growing in the West Indies. Resin is extracted from its wood, or chips of the wood can be boiled to make an infusion. It is used for joint pain and inflammation.

White Willow *Salix alba*
The bark is a source of salicin and from it comes salicylic acid from which aspirin was derived. Its extract therefore has a place in treating pain and inflammation just as aspirin has.

Wild Yam Dioscorea villosa

This is grown as a food in southern Africa and Asia as it has potato-like tubers containing starch. From it a steroid chemical can be extracted which was initially used as a source of oestrogen. It also has an anti-inflammatory effect useful in arthritis.

These and other herbal products are frequently used in combination as remedies for rheumatism and arthritis. One that has recently been tested and shown to have a significant effect in relieving the pain of osteoarthritis is *Reumalex*. This contains the following herbs: White Willow bark, Guaiacum Resin, Black Cohosh, Sarsaparilla and Poplar bark.

Homoeopathy

Homoeopathy is a system of medicine derived from the ancient Law of Similars This stated that the remedy for a complaint was to be found in a substance that would produce similar symptoms when given to a healthy person. Dr Samuel Hahnemann, an 18th century Leipzig physician, developed this principle. He made a large number of tests ("provings") on himself taking different substances and meticulously noting the symptoms that each produced, so building up a fund of knowledge of potential remedies appropriate to those symptoms.

Moreover, he found that a remedy could be made more powerful ("potentised") by being repeatedly diluted either tenfold or a hundredfold, as long as the solution was vigorously shaken ("succussed") at the time of each dilution. The resulting solution would be absorbed on to a small tablet of lactose, or on to granules, in which form it would retain its power indefinitely.

The modern homoeopathic practitioner still uses remedies prepared in this way. His full resources (materia medica) now have hundreds of remedies available in different potencies. Those used most often are the 6 and the 30 potencies, meaning that the mother tincture was diluted a hundredfold 6 times over, or 30 times over, and in some cases even more.

So detailed is the information available on each remedy that the practitioner can choose a treatment that matches not only the pattern of the patient's symptoms but also the nature of the patient himself. Consequently an appointment with a homoeopathic practitioner (who may or may not be medically qualified) is a lengthy affair: many questions are asked about the nature of the symptoms and also of the patient's character, likes and dislikes. After all this the appropriate remedy is selected.

Homoeopathic remedies that are on sale over the counter for self medication are usually of the 6 (centesimal) potency, which is relatively low. These offer a rather limited choice which, of course, is far less precise than having a detailed assessment made by an experienced homoeopathic practitioner, who has access to a wide range of possible remedies and potencies.

Some common remedies for rheumatism and arthritis that are available over the counter are as follows:

Rhus toxicodendron – for pain and stiffness which improves on movement.
Bryonia – for pain made worse by movement, and eased by rest and pressure.
Arnica – for pain in limbs or joints resulting from injury or bruising, even some time ago.
Pulsatilla – for muscular pains that shift from place to place.
Ruta – for pains in tendons, tendon sheaths & muscles.
Dulcamara – pains made worse by cold and damp.
Causticum – for pain improved by damp weather, and when there is a tendency to contracture.
Ledum – for muscle pains after stings, puncture wounds and injections.

For best effect a homoeopathic tablet should be held under the tongue until it has dissolved and no other strongly flavoured substance, or coffee or alcohol or drug should be taken at the same time. For acute symptoms up to 5 or 6 tablets should be taken at intervals of 15 to 30 minutes, otherwise 1 to 3 tablets may be taken at half hourly intervals. As in the case of herbal medicine homoeopathic treatments tend to act slowly and gently; they are free from toxic side effects which is an important reason for their appeal.

Acupuncture

Acupuncture is based on the ancient Chinese system of medicine and so has been in use in the Orient for hundreds, even thousands, of years, yet active interest in it in the West has only developed in the past 30 years.

There are now many practitioners of acupuncture in the UK, Europe and the USA who have undergone special training, sometimes in China itself, and some are also medically qualified.

The traditional Chinese teaching is that life energy – Ch'i or Qi – runs in the body in 12 invisible lines on each side of the body, the *meridians*. There are two further midline meridians, one at the front and one at the back. Each meridian runs partly within the body as well as just under the skin surface and all the internal organs feature on a meridian. Six of them run to or from the toes.

Disorders of health, which the Chinese physician may judge by the subtle art of pulse diagnosis, occur when the flow of Qi in one or more meridians is blocked. It is possible to correct this fault by stimulating the appropriate point on the relevant meridian by acupuncture or by moxibustion. Through long experience Chinese physicians have identified hundreds of such points.

The act of acupuncture involves the insertion of a fine sterilised steel needle into the correct point, to a depth of no more than a few millimetres and leaving it there for several minutes while the patient lies quietly relaxed. A number of needles may be inserted at the same time. A small added stimulus may be given by rotating a needle briefly, or by the passage of a weak electric current (electroacupuncture).

In *moxibustion* the therapist stimulates the acupuncture point by placing over it a small portion of a smouldering herb, usually mugwort *(Artemesia vulgaris)* or the smouldering tip of a moxa stick.

In *auricular acupuncture* the needle is inserted into one of many points on the ear which are believed to be connected to the rest of the body just as the meridians are.

Because of the wide ranging connections of the meridian system acupuncture can be used for many disorders, including psychological problems such as addictions to drugs or tobacco, eating disorders and obesity. There is ample evidence of its effectiveness in reports from Chine and from the West.

For *rheumatic disorders* acupuncture has been found helpful in treating back pain, cervical spondylosis, soft tissue rheumatism and rheumatoid arthritis. Acupuncture often makes it possible for drug dosages to be reduced, including steroid dosage.

Many *pain clinics* now make use of acupuncture. The neurologist's explanation of its effect is that the sensory stimulus from the needle may block or interfere with the passage of the pain signal to the brain ("gate theory"). It may also act by increasing the brain's secretion of natural pain blockers, the endorphins.

Acupressure is a simplified form of acupuncture suitable for self treatment. By applying firm finger pressure at points on the body similar to acupuncture points relief can be obtained from various types of pain and nausea. Books are available which explain the sites of these acupressure points (see Appendix).

Osteopathy

This is based on belief in the intimate relationship between bodily structure – principally of the spine – and bodily health. It recognises that the body's natural state is one of health and that all bodily systems will function better if any structural faults are sought and corrected.

The osteopathic practitioner undergoes a lengthy training comparable to that of a medical student, focussing on the musculoskeletal system in particular detail. He learns to examine a patient paying special attention to posture and movement, carefully sensing areas of stress in relation to muscles and joints. X rays are used as part of the examination.

Osteopathic treatment concentrates on manual manipulation of the spine at all levels and of the joints. In the process, the patient may feel or hear the "clicks" with which osteopathy is supposedly associated. In the USA osteopathy is practised as virtually a separate system of medicine, whereas in the UK it is associated primarily with manipulation techniques. In 1993 the Osteopathic Register was introduced.

The rheumatic condition for which osteopathy is mainly used is low back pain. Research studies have shown that osteopathy can produce better results than conventional treatments with rest, corsets, drugs and physiotherapy. It is also helpful in treating cervical spondylosis and many forms of soft tissue rheumatism. As a rule manipulation is followed up with a programme of exercises.

Chiropractic

The name "chiropractic" implies "treatment by the hands", meaning by a form of manipulation. Like osteopathy, it originated in the USA in the late 19th century, being originally based on the concept that all bodily disorders could be traced to a displaced vertebra – a belief long since discarded. Like osteopaths, chiropractors, whether in the USA or UK, undergo a detailed medical training, comparable to that of a doctor. They learn to enquire into a patient's medical history and to make a detailed medical examination.

Chiropractic treatment is based on manual manipulation, but with certain technical differences from osteopathy. It has been shown to be very effective in the treatment of back pain, spondylosis and soft tissue rheumatism.

Alexander method

F M Alexander was an Australian, born in 1869, who trained as an actor. However, he found that he had great difficulty with hoarseness and was unable to project his voice as an actor should. There seemed to be no medical explanation for this, so he set out on a long process of self observation. He discovered that unconscious muscle tensions and faults of posture and of breathing were really the cause of the incorrect use of his larynx. Having become aware of these faults he was able to relearn the use of his body with particular reference to posture, movement, breathing and voice production.

When other actors asked him for help he found that he could only assist them by working with each person on a one-to-one basis, using his hands to sense the areas of muscle tension and to guide them to a better use of the body.

The Alexander method is now taught world-wide by specially trained teachers, who work individually with each patient just as Alexander himself did. It is seen as a learning process and not as a therapy, for each person has to relearn the habits of posture and movement, even though they may have seemed right previously. A number of one-to-one sessions are necessary. The method is particularly appreciated by actors, musicians and public speakers. It is valuable in correcting the faults which underlie forms of soft tissue rheumatism and is of help too in cases of established arthritis.

Other complementary therapies

Of the many other forms of complementary medicine a number can be of help, directly or indirectly, to the sufferer from rheumatism or arthritis.

Relief of stress. Stress can be an important cause of muscle tension, postural faults and fatigue, so contributing to some forms of soft tissue rheumatism. With any kind of established arthritis, stress and anxiety make symptoms and disability harder to bear. *Massage* helps relieve pain and tension, and is now used more as a complementary than as a conventional therapy. It may be combined with *aromatherapy* in which a wide range of essential oils are used, each having its own qualities and indications. Many trained therapists are available throughout the UK. The Japanese technique of *shiatsu* is related to the principles of acupuncture and Chinese medicine. While the patient reclines and relaxes on a mattress on the floor the therapist works progressively over the body, applying gentle but firm pressure at selected points using her hands and arms.

Relaxation sessions for patients either singly or in groups can be a valuable source of support in many forms of disease in which anxiety is an element. In a number of cancer clinics tuition is now given in relaxation, sometimes combined with *meditation* and *visualisation* of the body's healing powers. These approaches can be equally supportive for patients with arthritis.

Self healing. As a rule we fail to appreciate the power of the body to heal itself from disease and to overcome disability. Meir Schneider began by learning to overcome his own severe visual disabilities and progressed to helping others with eye problems, with neuromuscular disorders (some with no known effective orthodox treatment) and arthritis. The techniques that he and his followers teach are based on physical and postural exercises, undertaken with full awareness of the mind controlling the body.

Healing. There are some thousands of men and women healers in the UK. A minority are associated with religious organisations or may be ordained ministers themselves, but most are non denominational. Most are recognised members of the National Federation of Spiritual Healers, the Confederation of Healing Organisations or other bodies: this means that they are committed to agreed ethical standards of practice. A number of healers now work in co-operation with doctors. Many people with serious health problems such as arthritis find that sessions with a healer give them an inner strength with helps their recovery.

Conclusion

The relationship between complementary and conventional medicine is the subject of national and European debate. Co-operation between the two is likely to grow, largely because the public wishes that this should be so. The medical reaction, naturally, is to require evidence that complementary therapies are effective, that their practitioners should have adequate training and that they should maintain professional standards of practice. To some extent there is approval within the NHS in that certain therapies – osteopathy, acupuncture and homoeopathy – can be provided at NHS expense if a GP requests them. This is good news for the patient with rheumatism or arthritis. In some cases it may prove to be economically effective, i.e. less costly, in the long run than conventional treatment. Even so, many patients will no doubt continue their present practice of independently seeking self help through herbal remedies, massage, sessions with healers and other forms of complementary medicine.

11 | Appendix

Helpful Organisations and Books

Registered charities concerned with Rheumatism

1. *The Arthritic Association*
First Floor Suite, 2 Hyde Gardens, Eastbourne, East Sussex BN21 4PN.
Ref DJC. The Association provides information and assistance for the
home treatment of Arthritis and aims to promote and finance research
into its causes and treatment.

2. *Arthritis & Rheumatism Council*
Copeman House, St Mary's Court, St Mary's Gate, Chesterfield,
Derbyshire S41 7TD.
Generously funds medical and scientific research into rheumatism.
Supports medical teaching in rheumatology. Provides free information
pamphlets on rheumatism and arthritis to the public.

3. *Arthritis Care*
18 Stephenson Way, London NW1 2HD.
Helps and informs people with arthritis. Has Regional organisations and
a section for Young Arthritis care. Publishes quarterly "Arthritis News"
costing £5 p.a.

4. *National Osteoporosis Society*
Director Linda Edwards, PO Box 10, Radstock, Bath BA3 3YB.
Provides information and advice on osteoporosis to the public and to
doctors.

5. *National Back Pain Association*
16 Elm Tree Road, Teddington, Middlesex TW11 8ST.
Promotes research on the causes and treatment of back pain.

6. *National Ankylosing Spondylitis Association (NASS)*
Director Fergus Rogers, 3 Grosvenor Crescent, London SW1X 7ER.
Provides information to patients and to doctors, promotes research into
Ankylosing Spondylitis.

7. *Psoriatic Arthropathy Alliance*
136 High St, Bushey, Herts. WD2 3DJ.
Supports and informs patients with psoriatic arthritis.

8. *Lupus UK*
51 North St, Romford, Essex RM1 3BA.
Supports and informs patients with Systemic Lupus.

9. *Raynaud's and Scleroderma Association*
112 Crewe Road, Alsager, Cheshire ST7 2JA.
Supports and informs patients with these complaints.

10. *Primary Care Rheumatology Society*
P O Box 42, Northallerton, N Yorks DL7 8YG.
Informs and promotes postgraduate training of GPs in rheumatology.

11. *Institute of Complementary Medicine*
P O Box 194, Tavern Quay, London SE16 1QZ.
Will provide information on qualified practitioners of various forms of
complementary medicine.

12. *National Federation of Spiritual Healers*
Old Manor Farm Studio, Church St, Sunbury on Thames, Middlesex
TW16 6RG. Tel: 019327.83164.
On telephone enquiry will provide information on registered healers in
different parts of the country.

Books

1. *The New Natural Family Doctor*
Editor Dr Andrew Stanway, Gaia Books Ltd, London.
A well produced introduction to healthy living with clear summaries of many forms of complementary medicine and their application in many complaints.

2. *Lets Eat Right to Keep Fit*
Adelle Davis, Thorsons, London.
A very readable racy introduction to healthy nutrition.

3. *Diet for life: a cookbook for arthritics*
Mary Laver & Margaret Smith, Pan Books, London.
A dietary guide and cookbook written by a sufferer from rheumatoid arthritis for whom the Dong diet worked.

4. *Arthritis at Your Age*
Jill Holroyd, Grindleton Press, P O Box 222, Ipswich IP9 2TX.
A sympathetic and informative handbook for the teenager or young adult with arthritis.

5. *Self Healing: My Life and Vision*
Meir Schneider, Arkana Books, London.
An impressive account of what can be done to promote our own healing and recovery.

6. *Overcoming Rheumatism and Arthritis*
Phyllis Speight, C W Daniel Co Ltd, Saffron Walden, Essex.
Homeopathic remedies described by an experienced practitioner.

7. *The New Holistic Herbal*
David Hoffmann, Element Books, Shaftesbury, Dorset.
A comprehensive account of herbal medicines and their uses.

OTHER BOOKS FROM AMBERWOOD PUBLISHING ARE:

Aromatherapy – A Guide for Home Use by Christine Westwood. All you need to know about essential oils and using them. £1.99.

Aromatherapy – For Stress Management by Christine Westwood. Covering the use of essential oils for everyday stress-related problems. £2.99.

Aromatherapy – For Healthy Legs and Feet by Christine Westwood. A comprehensive guide to the use of essential oils for the treatment of legs and feet, including illustrated massage instructions. £2.99.

Aromatherapy – Simply For You by Marion Del Gaudio Mak. A clear, simple and comprehensive guide to Aromatherapy for beginners. £1.99.

Aromatherapy – A Nurses Guide by Ann Percival SRN. This book draws on the author's medical skills and experience as a qualified aromatherapist to provide the ultimate, safe, lay guide to the natural benefits of Aromatherapy. Including recipes and massage techniques for many medical conditions and a quick reference chart. £2.99.

Aromatherapy – A Nurses Guide for Women by Ann Percival SRN. Building on the success of her first 'Nurses Guide', this book concentrates on women's health for all ages. Including sections on PMT, menopause, infertility, cellulite. Everything a woman needs to know about healthcare using aromatherapy. £2.99.

Aroma Science – The Chemistry & Bioactivity of Essential Oils by Dr Maria Lis-Balchin. With a comprehensive list of the Oils and scientific analysis – a must for all with an interest in the science of Aromatherapy. Includes sections on methodology, the sense of smell and the history of Aromatherapy. £4.99.

Plant Medicine – A Guide for Home Use (New Edition) by Charlotte Mitchell MNIMH. A guide to home use giving an insight into the wonderful healing qualities of plants. £2.99.

Woman Medicine – Vitex Agnus Castus by Simon Mills MA, FNIMH. The wonderful story of the herb that has been used for centuries in the treatment of women's problems. £2.99.

Ancient Medicine – Ginkgo Biloba (New Edition) by Dr Desmond Corrigan BSc(Pharms), MA, Phd, FLS, FPSI. Improved memory, circulation and concentration are associated in this book with medicine from this fascinating tree. £2.99.

Indian Medicine – The Immune System by Dr Desmond Corrigan BSc(Pharms), MA, Phd, FLS, FPSI. An intriguing account of the history and science of the plant called Echinacea and its power to influence the immune system. £2.99.

Herbal Medicine for Sleep & Relaxation by Dr Desmond Corrigan BSc(Pharms), MA, PhD, FLS, FPSI. An expertly written guide to the natural sedatives as an alternative to orthodox drug therapies, drawing on the latest medical research, presented in an easy reference format. £2.99.

Herbal First Aid by Andrew Chevallier BA, MNIMH. A beautifully clear reference book of natural remedies and general first aid in the home. £2.99.

Natural Taste – Herbal Teas, A Guide for Home Use by Andrew Chevallier BA, MNIMH. This charmingly illustrated book contains a comprehensive compendium of Herbal Teas gives information on how to make it, its benefits, history and folklore. £2.99.

Garlic– How Garlic Protects Your Heart by Prof E. Ernst MD, PhD. Used as a medicine for over 4500 years, this book examines the latest scientific evidence supporting Garlic's effect in reducing cardiovascular disease, the Western World's number one killer. £3.99.

Insomnia – Doctor I Can't Sleep by Dr Adrian Williams FRCP. Written by one of the world's leading sleep experts, Dr Williams explains the phenomenon of sleep and sleeping disorders and gives advice on treatment. With 25% of the adult population reporting difficulties sleeping – this book will be essential reading for many. £2.99.

Signs & Symptoms of Vitamin Deficiency by Dr Leonard Mervyn BSc, PhD, C.Chem, FRCS. A home guide for self diagnosis which explains and assesses Vitamin Therapy for the prevention of a wide variety of diseases and illnesses. £2.99.

Causes & Prevention of Vitamin Deficiency by Dr Leonard Mervyn BSc, PhD, C.Chem, FRCS. A home guide to the Vitamin content of foods and the depletion caused by cooking, storage and processing. It includes advice for those whose needs are increased due to lifestyle, illness etc. £2.99.

Eyecare Eyewear – For Better Vision by Mark Rossi Bsc, MBCO. A complete guide to eyecare and eyewear including an assessment of the types of spectacles and contact lenses available and the latest corrective surgical procedures. £3.99.